SPRINGER SERIES ON INDUSTRY AND HEALTH CARE
NUMBER 1

Payer, Provider, Consumer: Industry Confronts Health Care Costs

Diana Chapman Walsh
Richard H. Egdahl

Springer-Verlag   New York Heidelberg Berlin

Springer Series on Industry and Health Care
Richard H. Egdahl, M.D., Ph.D.
Center for Industry and Health Care
Boston University Health Policy Institute
53 Bay State Road
Boston, Massachusetts 02215

Library of Congress Cataloging in Publication Data

Main entry under title:

Payer, provider, consumer.

    (Springer series on industry and health care; no. 1)
    Includes bibliographical references.
    1. Medical care, Cost of—United States—Congresses. 2. Labor and
laboring classes—Medical care—United States—Congresses. 3. Insurance
Health—United States—Congresses. I. Walsh, Diana Chapman.
II. Egdahl, Richard Harrison. [1. Costs and cost analysis. 2. Industry
3. Health services. 4. Insurance, Health. W1 SP685 no. 1/W74 W224p]
RA410.53.P37   338.4'3   77-21020

Printed in the United States of America.

9 8 7 6 5 4 3 2 1

ISBN 0-387-90295-3 Springer-Verlag New York Heidelberg Berlin
ISBN 3-540-90295-3 Springer-Verlag Berlin Heidelberg New York

Preface

With this first monograph, Springer-Verlag launches an unusual publishing venture. The purpose of the Springer Series on Industry and Health Care is to explore in depth the current and potential future role of industry—both management and labor in all private sector enterprises—as a financer of health care benefits, as a provider of health care services, and as an extremely influential "consumer" of health care.

The assumption behind the series is that private industry has the capability, as an alternative to increased government intervention, to effect major change in the health care delivery system and is beginning to show evidence of exercising that influence. The subject matter covered by the series crosses boundaries between disciplines and specialities—occupational medicine, medical care, public health, economics, business administration, law, public policy, medical sociology—and arises in disparate arenas—labor–management relations, corporate negotiations with insurance carriers, physician–patient interactions, public policy, and politics.

The Springer Series will draw much of its material from interdisciplinary working conferences, will analyze and synthesize the discussions, add timely background material, and be published within no more than six months of the conferences on which they build. The series will consist of four monographs a year and two volumes of background papers.

This first monograph examines industry's various roles in health care, as payer, provider, and consumer. The second and third, a book and a monograph, will delve deeper into the problems and prospects of industry's changing role in the delivery of health services.

Intended to serve in part as a road map through future volumes of the series, this first monograph draws on a greater variety of sources—two different conferences and a partial review of recent literature—than will future monographs. One conference was held in Ithaca, New York, in early May 1977 under the aegis of Cornell University's Sloan Program of Hospital and Health Services Administration. Entitled "Strategies for Controlling Medical Care Costs," the program was the first of a series Cornell intends to hold for business executives concerned with health care issues. We are grateful to Cornell's Graduate School of Business and Public Administration and to Douglas R. Brown, the director of Cornell's Health Program for Business Executives, for consenting to our using portions of that conference as a core of subject matter for this monograph.

The second conference from which this monograph draws was sponsored by the Boston University Health Policy Institute, aided by a grant from the Robert Wood Johnson Foundation. Held in Boston in early June 1977, it was entitled "Industry-Sponsored Health Programs," and consisted of a day and a half of discussion, with specially prepared background papers distributed in advance of the conference to the participants. The contributions of the June conference will be captured more fully in the next two issues of the series. Quotations in this monograph that are not otherwise identified come from one of the two conferences; information by which to identify the speakers is included in the appendix.

It is our hope that the entire series will be useful in both industry and health spheres, to all who are interested in health services delivery, health planning, prepaid health plans, occupational medicine, the cost-quality equation in health care, and the financing of health services. Different segments of this diverse audience will doubtless have varying reactions to and uses for the material included here. Employee benefit managers may find the payer section most relevant, occupational health professionals and others interested in medical care may gravitate to the provider section, and health planning proponents to the consumer section. We have tried to include enough background information in each section to facilitate and indeed encourage crossing over by interested readers into areas outside their major sphere of concern.

A final caveat may be in order. In the interest of getting this monograph out reasonably quickly, we naturally had to make some compromises—forgoing one more search through the literature, a few more outside reviews, another working draft or two. Difficult as they were, we are comfortable with these trade-offs for we do not view this first product as the definitive word on industry and health care. It is but an opening statement in an ongoing discussion. Many problems and issues remain to be addressed and ultimately resolved, but we feel it is critically important to get the discussion under way.

And a final word of thanks. We are indebted to the Washington Business Group on Health for advice and assistance in arranging our conference, and to its director, Willis B. Goldbeck, for his help with the conference and for a valuable critical review of an early draft of this monograph. Substantial improvements resulted also from the numerous suggestions of William J. Bicknell, Medical Director of the United Mine Workers of America Health and Retirement Funds and an ongoing consultant to the Boston University Health

Policy Institute's Program in Industry and Health Care. Members of the Health Policy Institute staff have been helpful and we thank them, in particular: John Friedland for a very careful reading of a draft and a number of valuable suggestions, and Mark Schofield for help with the library research. We are grateful also to the participants in the two conferences from which we drew material. Whether quoted or not, everyone who spoke up at those conferences contributed to whatever insights we were able to bring to this subject. The final product, of course, is entirely our responsibility.

Boston,
August 1977

Richard H. Egdahl
Series Editor

Diana Chapman Walsh
Assistant Editor

Contents

Introduction: Industry Confronts Health Care Costs

1

Through industry's window onto the health care system it is possible to see most of the urgent policy choices confronting us, along with many of the built-in conflicts that confound those choices:

How much money does society wish to channel into health care and by implication away from other goals?

How do we reconcile the need to curtail runaway increases in health care costs with problems of unmet needs and uneven distribution of resources?

Where do the scales tip between uniform quality and maximal efficiency?

Where on the continuum shall we stop between a pluralistic, decentralized, and undisciplined system on one side and a monolithic, regulated, and involuntary one on the other?

What payoffs can we reasonably expect from health services, what is a reasonable price for them, and how do we judge whether we are getting our money's worth?

While payers, providers, and consumers have strong and often counter-vailing interests in these questions, industry wears, at various times, all three mantles. We are defining industry broadly to include both management and labor in all private-sector business enterprises. As a payer for health care on a large and growing scale through employee benefit packages, industry has vital interests that are tightly bound up with the nation's need to slow the rise of health care costs. As a provider of care through diverse in-house programs and clinics, industry faces dilemmas of accountability, confidentiality, and evalua-tion, along with expanded responsibilities for the health and welfare of work-ers. As a consumer of health care whose potential influence in the system derives in part from the massive numbers of workers who use health care services, industry has an opportunity and perhaps an obligation to share its expertise as well as to learn by participating in community efforts to find equitable ways to allocate limited resources and improve the quality of the health care system.

The division between the payer and the consumer role is somewhat arbitrary, but is made at the point where industry becomes involved in commu-nity health activities independently of an obligation—already proffered and accepted—to finance specific health services through the benefit package. For example, some firms have assigned an executive with no responsibility for employee benefits to spend most or all of his time dealing with community health issues. A person such as this is clearly performing a function that is broader than the traditional payer role. In the past, industry has usually preferred to avoid direct involvement with the delivery of health care outside the plant and is still reluctant to become deeply embroiled in the issue of quality of care. But growing financial participation is forcing a new look at how the money is spent.

The 1970s have seen an upsurge of public interest in private industry's influence and obligations in the health care arena. Whether as payer, provider, or consumer, industry has for many years played an important but not a central role in the health care system: few of industry's current and potential roles are new. But the intensity with which they are being played is greater, the oppor-tunities for impact are wider, the stakes are higher, and the political timetable appears shorter.

So concluded the President's Council on Wage and Price Stability after a year-long investigation of rising health care costs, completed in 1976. The council held open hearings in New York, Chicago, San Francisco, Philadel-phia, Houston, and Miami, heard testimony from diverse points of view, and published a final report that described ongoing private sector efforts to contain health care costs and challenged the private sector to "step up its efforts manyfold."[1] The council's visibility and the information it generated inspired a succession of derivative reports in the mass media. Some of the material presented here on employer involvement in health care also draws on the council's findings, supplemented by substantial updating by the Washington Business Group on Health.[2]

Industry's stepped-up involvement in the health care system can be traced to a variety of forces. First, the Occupational Safety and Health Act (OSHA) of 1970 has certainly had an impact. Establishing a "general duty" on the part of all industry to provide a safe working environment, the act created the Occupational Safety and Health Administration which has been mandating specific environmental standards as well as medical surveillance of workers exposed to certain substances. At a minimum, the act has enhanced awareness within management and labor of the need for programs to reduce exposure to potential agents of occupational injury and disease. Its passage in turn reflected other conditions: an apparent increase in rates of occupational injury and a general awakening to the pervasiveness of occupational disease, technological change in the workplace calling for more sophisticated safeguards to health, the emergence of the ecology movement with its emphasis on the ill effects of environmental pollution, and the altered character of the work force, with more education and higher wages, accompanied by a broader set of expectations and demands.[3] The influence of OSHA on industry-sponsored health programs is considered in chapter 3 which describes industry's role as provider of care.

Second, industry's expanding roles are both cause and effect of a rising demand for health services. The relationship of employment-related financing arrangements to elevated demand and spiraling costs is a central theme in industry's role as payer for care, and is elaborated in chapter 2.

Third, the emergence of the health industry as the largest industry in the country in terms of employees, and the third largest in income produced,[4] carries implications for all private industry: for management's commitment to the free enterprise system in the face of increasing government financing and regulation of health care, and the chance that the system may ultimately be "nationalized"; for labor's concern over employment and the reality that the health delivery system serves important economic functions quite apart from the delivery of medical care. It provides jobs for a wide range of occupations from physicians, nurses, and administrators to clerks, aides, and orderlies— some 4.5 million workers in all.[4] Hospitals and other health facilities are economic assets in many communities. Rick J. Carlson, who has been a vocal critic of the health care system, wonders if its chief redeeming virtue may in fact be the provision of jobs:

> The most perceptive and most useful way to look at the health care system is, first and foremost, as an employer. In fact, I can say without too much whimsy that it wouldn't bother me overly if we spent 12 percent of our gross national product on the health system, so long as it gainfully employed a substantial number of people, everybody very merrily, happily doing what they were doing. As long as we didn't indulge in the rhetoric that the investment had much to do with health.

NATIONAL HEALTH EXPENDITURES AND PERCENTAGE OF GROSS NATIONAL PRODUCT

Year	Billions of Dollars	Percentage of GNP	Dollars per Capita
1990		10–12 (projected)	
1976	139.3	8.6	638
1975	118.5	8.3	564
1974	104.2	7.7	498
1973	94.2	7.7	463
1972	86.4	7.8	425
1971	77.2	7.6	386
1970	69.2	7.2	350
1966	42.1	5.9	225
1965	38.9	5.9	205
1960	25.9	5.2	142
1950	12.0	4.6	82
1940	3.9	4.1	30
1929	3.6	3.6	29

Sources: Past levels from U.S. Department of Health, Education, and Welfare: *Health in the United States 1975: A Chartbook* (Rockville, Md.: DHEW pub. no. [HRA] 76-1233, 1976), p. 6. Projection From Executive Office of the President, Council on Wage and Price Stability: *The Complex Puzzle of Rising Health Care Costs* (Washington, D.C.: USGPO no. 052–003–00255–8, December 1976), pp. 77, 93.

But the first imperative is cost control. It is now widely known that health care costs have been increasing much faster than other prices, and are involving a growing share of gross national product: from 5.9 percent in 1965 to an unprecedented 8.6 percent in 1976, with 10 to 12 percent forecast as a distinct possibility by 1990 (see box).[5] Health care expenditures have tripled since 1965 and are believed, by the Council on Wage and Price Stability, to be an important factor contributing to the overall rate of inflation in the economy. It is inaccurate—but not uncommon—to assume the obverse and dismiss rising health care costs as a mere symptom of general inflation. The reasons for rising expenditures are the subject of considerable debate, but it is known that they reflect some combination of increases in price, in the use of services, and in their dimensions or quality. Population growth, too, is a contributing factor.

The effects of this cost spiral are being felt by industry. Insurance premiums for employee health benefits are increasing at a rate of at least 10 percent each year (see box). Health care is now a major payroll item, a central issue at the bargaining table, and a serious drain on the average worker's

INDUSTRY'S RISING HEALTH CARE COSTS

Flux in benefits and beneficiary groups makes it difficult for large, multiple-site firms to isolate the costs of health insurance per se. Recent estimates, however, have placed the annual cost increase at 10 to 12 percent, perhaps higher, with no change in benefits.[a] Specific firms have reported the following trends in health insurance costs. These are offered simply as illustrations and are not a valid basis for comparisons from one company to another.

Alcoa:	1974–1975 increase of 23.9%, with no major benefit changes.[b]
Bethlehem Steel:	1970: $48 million or $371 per employee; 1976: $371 million or $1,069 per employee.[a]
Continental Bank:	1971–1975 Per employee cost increase at five Chicago locations of 45 percent, apart from benefit changes.[a]
Continental Illinois Corporation:	Per employee cost: 1971—$326, 1976—$535, 1977—$556.[c]
Eastern Airlines:	Per employee cost: 1973—$430, 1976—$850 (est.) Annual increase of 25%; no other cost element, save fuel, has escalated as rapidly.[a]
General Motors:	1976—$825 million,[a] 1977—$1.3 billion.[b]
Rohm and Haas:	1970–1976 increase of 90–120% or 11–13% per year.[a]
FMC:[d]	1974–1975: 37.2% increase; 1975–1976: 32% increase.[b]

a. Council on Wage and Price Stability: *The Complex Puzzle of Rising Health Care Costs* (Washington, D.C.: USGPO no. 052–003–00255–8, December 1976).

b. Washington Business Group on Health: "Private Sector Perspective on the Problems of Health Care Costs, working paper, April 1977.

c. *Employee Benefit Plan Review*, Chicago, June 1977.

budget (see figures 1–3). Health care accounted for about 40 percent of fringe benefits in 1974, a fourfold increase over 1950.[6]

However, cost control is but one of several imperatives. Willis B. Goldbeck, Director of the Washington Business Group on Health, relates the cost imperative to other national goals: "Just as surely as we cannot create major new national health initiatives without first controlling the costs, so too we cannot have a health system of adequate quality and public acceptance if the whole focus is on cost control. Therein lies the challenge."[7] The issue then is not simply costs per se but the companion question—and one that business can easily relate to—of "return on investment": the duplication and waste said to exist in the system, the insufficient planning, the distorted financial incentives. These are problems that private industry is eminently qualified to address.

Richard M. Martin, of Goodyear Tire & Rubber, argues that the corporate sector has been slow to make the necessary commitment:

> We really should slap ourselves on the wrist for what we haven't done. With sufficient corporate commitment, there's a great deal we can do, and first of all we must address waste. I firmly believe that if all of us—the government and the private sector—elimi-

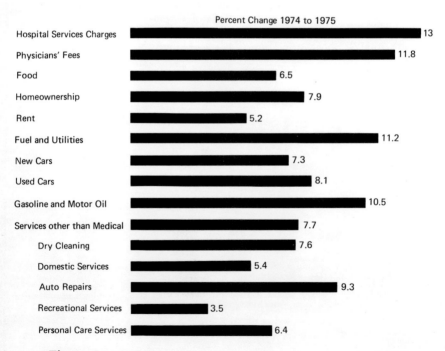

Figure 1.

Rates of price increase: health care vs. other goods and services, 1974–1975. *Source:* Council on Wage and Price Stability: *The Complex Puzzle of Rising Health Care Costs* (Washington, D.C.: USGPO, December 1976), p. 75.

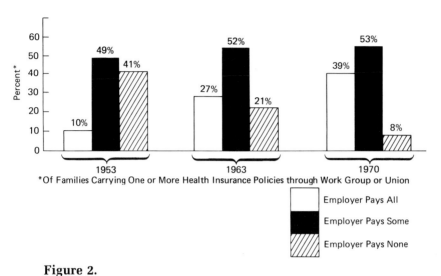

Figure 2.

Employer participation in the payment for health insurance. *Source:* U.S. Department of Health, Education, and Welfare: *Health U.S., 1975*, p. 61, table A-27.

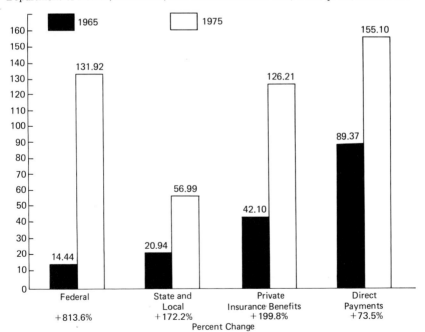

Figure 3.

Per capita expenditures for personal health care. *Source:* Council on Wage and Price Stability: *The Complex Puzzle of Rising Health Care Costs* (Washington, D.C.: USGPO, December 1976), p. 72.

*nated the out-and-out, obvious waste in the health care system, we
would be a long way toward controlling or at least stabilizing costs.*

The waste in the system of which Martin and others speak is only obliquely
attributable to mismanagement within health care facilities or services. Sometimes it is due to insufficient or faulty long-range planning—as, for example,
when a hospital accepts a financing package for a capital construction project
that is more expensive than need be. But usually, the "waste" alleged in the
system is a result of overlapping and redundant facilities, equipment, or
services within an area or region. These issues are discussed in more detail in
chapter 4.

The organizing theme of this monograph, which stands as both an
overview and a preview of future volumes in this series, is that industry is a key
participant in the health sector in three roles: as payer, provider, and consumer.
Any attempt to classify so complex a subject is naturally fraught with difficulty.
A virtue of this particular conceptual scheme is not only its simplicity, but the
message it telegraphs: industry is *already* deeply enmeshed in the health care
system. Of course, the scheme requires arbitrary separations that are often
simply questions of degree or emphasis, and sometimes fails to work. For
example, prospective reimbursement of hospitals and second opinion programs for elective surgery are ways for companies to contain the cost of the
benefit package, and are thus treated here as an aspect of industry's role as
payer. However, such programs may also have broader implications for the
delivery system and may be among the contributions industry can make as an
informed and influential consumer of health care, capable of using its buying
power to persuade the insurance carriers of the need for changes in the design
and administration of benefit packages. Similarly, prepaid health plans and
preventive programs can be viewed in all three categories. All such classification depends on the context of the particular program and how global or
circumscribed its underlying objectives happen to be, but classification is
useful in spite of its artificiality.

And that raises another issue. Industry is heterogeneous. Here, as already
suggested, we are defining the term broadly, to subsume both management and
labor in all private-sector economic activity, including agriculture, forestry and
fisheries, mining, construction, manufacturing, transportation, communication, and public utilities, wholesale and retail trade, finance, insurance, and
real estate, service establishments, and professional and related services.[8]
Generalization about roles played by such disparate organizations is hazardous. The size of the industry or firm comes into play, as do its geographical
location, the composition of its work force, how it is managed and structured,
what it produces and how. Size may be the cardinal factor, as suggested by the
AFL-CIO's Sheldon Samuels, who asserts that there are "tens of thousands of
small companies that have no health program, want none, and should not be
given any."[9] But while the larger firms and unions will continue to break the
new ground, there is no reason to doubt that smaller ones can, through a
process of consolidation and cooperation, build on the foundations that have
been laid. And even within the largest entities, inherent conflicts of policy and

divergent incentives at different levels of the organization can dilute the advantages of size. Such conflicts are most easily envisaged in situations where a corporation committed to some health goal (perhaps health promotion or community health planning) also produces a product that is antithetical to that goal (cigarettes, or a high-cost technological medical device that may be overutilized).

Other conflicts are equally near the surface: the resentment that can be anticipated if there is a retrenchment on employee health benefits; the labor-management disputes that have punctuated the occupational health and safety movement; contention about the accountability of the plant physician and his ability or desire to preserve the confidentiality of his patients' records; the political voltage that will be generated if the health planning process really begins to close down duplicative facilities.

As private industry comes to grips with its role vis-à-vis the health care system, these and related issues will almost certainly be addressed. Whether and how they are resolved will map the future of the health care delivery system.

Industry as Payer: Employee Health Benefits

2

Of the three capacities in which industry can influence the medical marketplace, the role of payer or purchasing agent is perhaps the most complex. Yet industry as payer is a logical place to start, in part because it is here that industry feels the direct impact of rising health care costs, in part because some economists attribute to this role fundamental problems that are causing costs to rise. The history of industry's role as payer for health care demonstrates without doubt that over the years management and labor have profoundly affected the organization and financing of the health care delivery system, often more by chance than by design.

Assuming a Broader Role

Sown in the early 1900s with the introduction of commercial group health insurance to replace lost income for victims of specified illnesses, the seeds of the present financing system germinated slowly at first. By 1930 only about 2 percent of the labor force was enrolled in health or disability insurance programs,[1] which still emphasized replacement of lost income.[2] Into this desultory market entered Blue Cross, at first inspired less by the needs of patients than by the pressing plight of hospitals. Between 1929 and 1930, the Depression had cut the average receipts per patient in the nation's hospitals from $200 to under $60, had reduced the average occupancy from 71 to 64 percent, and had already led to deep deficits with worse in prospect.[3] The pattern for Blue Cross was set at Baylor University Hospital in Texas, where, in 1929, 1,250 school teachers each began prepaying 50¢ a month to cover up to twenty-one days of care a year in that hospital. Recognizing in prepayment a device to secure a stable funding base, the hospital system threw its resources and expertise behind the innovation and succeeded in the early 1930s in creating or helping to create thirty-nine local Blue Cross plans.

From its inception, health insurance focused on coverage of hospital care, which has persisted as the most widely held and best covered benefit. Of those first Blue Cross plans, twenty-two were funded entirely by local hospitals and five were partially so.[4] Through the 1930s and beyond, local hospitals and the American Hospital Association are said to have sought and acquired considerable control over the individual Blue Cross plans and the national Blue Cross Association.[5] The plans may have owed their early success to guarantees by participating hospitals to exempt subscribers from financial obligation for bills an insolvent Blue Cross plan might be unable to pay. By 1938, thirty-eight Blue Cross plans had enrolled 1.4 million Americans, in contrast to only 100,000 participants in private hospital insurance plans. The first Blue Shield plan was established in 1939 to cover medical and surgical services, as distinct from hospitalization.

World War II was a watershed. While wartime price stabilization regulations contained wage increases, fringe benefits were exempted in the belief that they would not fuel inflation. As part of the collective bargaining of an expanding union movement, health insurance came to be a supplement to income rather than a protection against untoward risk.[6]

Up to this point, the labor movement had been pursuing a relatively independent course. Early craft unions and a few industrial unions (notably the International Ladies' Garment Workers Union) had financed health and welfare benefits through union dues.[7] In some cases these "sick benefit funds" were among the organization's most attractive services to its members.[8] Prior to the postwar labor push for fringe benefits, some employers had unilaterally established health and welfare plans. During the war, the United Mine Workers of America (UMWA) staged a long and bruising strike which culminated in the Krug–Lewis Agreement establishing a Welfare and Retirement Fund. Today the renamed UMWA Health and Retirement Funds are in many ways the prototype Taft–Hartley trust, now providing through a multiemployer, joint labor-management fund health and pension benefits to over 800,000 coal miners, retired and disabled miners, and their dependents living in forty-nine states. In 1976 the funds paid out almost $225 million for health care for the covered population that year.[9]

Immediately after the war, labor rallied behind the second of many political efforts on behalf of national health insurance (the first had occurred without organized labor's support after World War I), but returned to the push for fringe benefits when the national campaign fizzled. Unions representing the steel, auto, electrical, transportation, communications, and building and service industries followed the United Mine Workers' lead, and by 1958 about 14 million union members and another 22 million dependents (some 29 percent of all health plan enrollees) were covered by plans that had been collectively negotiated. This relatively small percentage of the total provided nonetheless the basis for the far-reaching influence that collectively negotiated plans do have, often paving the way for shifts and innovations in the scope and structure of the employee benefit package of both union and nonunion employees. One can speculate that this influence derives sometimes from an anticipatory reaction on the part of nonunionized employers hoping to avoid unionization.

Typically, the Taft-Hartley trusts (some 4,800 plans in 1973, representing less than 4 percent of all group health insurance plans) exist in multiemployer situations, for example in service, coal mining, construction, apparel, and casual employment.[10] The most common pattern of bargaining in these cases is to negotiate prospectively, for the duration of the collective bargaining agreement, a fixed contribution from the signatory companies (usually a certain number of cents per hour, a set percentage of the payroll or an amount reflecting rates of productivity, such as coal tonnage in the mining industry). The level of income to the fund is thus determined by the wage agreement, and unanticipated expenses or shortages in expected contributions can force cuts in the benefit package. For example, the trustees of the United Mine Workers' Health and Retirement Fund, operating under the terms of a contract that continues until December 6, 1977, were forced in June 1977 to institute significant cost-sharing (coinsurance and deductibles) by beneficiaries because of flagging productivity and consequent reductions in employer contributions. Certainly labor feels stronger incentives to control health care costs in plans with a finite employer contribution than in those where the employment contract guarantees a certain level of benefits regardless of cost.

Single-employer plans and large manufacturing unions tend to negotiate a fixed level of benefits rather than a dollar amount. Management sometimes prefers this approach because it involves the company in determining the level of coverage, allows it to shop for cost-efficient benefits, and to reap the consequent savings if there are any.[11] The reverse, of course, is also true so that the stronger incentive to hold down costs in this case is the company's rather than the workers'. Unions complain that information on costs is withheld from them in fixed cost agreements and argue that such information must be shared if cooperative efforts to control costs are to succeed.[12]

During the 1940s and 1950s, driven by the push for fringe benefits, health insurance expanded into the newly opened market. The health insurance industry is thus relatively new and in most cases is a secondary line of business engrafted on by much older life insurance companies. Major medical coverage designed to help finance a spectrum of health services was introduced during the late 1940s. Until 1966—when Medicare and Medicaid radically altered the market for health insurance by enlisting many Blue Cross and Blue Shield organizations and some commercial underwriters as fiscal intermediaries for the government—the growth of the private carriers usually outpaced that of the Blues, because of structural and operating differences endowing commercial carriers with a slight competitive edge in negotiating contracts with large employers and employee groups. Time and competition have worn thin those original distinctions, but they need to be recognized as part of the context underlying the current system.

At the beginning Blue Cross was committed to community rating, whereby a uniform premium is set for all potential members without regard for actuarily determined differences in risk, as perhaps for the infirm or the elderly members of a group. Most of the commercial carriers tend to see health coverage as an adjunct to other lines of insurance (group life, disability, workmen's compensation), and they saw an opportunity to use actuarial data to set premiums by experience rating. This approach enabled them to offer employers and union groups substantially lower premiums than those based on community rates. Blue Cross was compelled gradually to abandon its community rating system rather than to be left to insure only groups and individuals self-selected for their adverse risk. In a sense, then, the fringe benefit push of organized labor can be blamed for driving out the community rating system[13] and creating a situation in which the government ultimately had to intervene to cover the groups who were unable under the experience rating system to secure reasonably priced health insurance coverage.[14]

From the outset the individual Blue Cross and Blue Shield plans and their national associations were designated nonprofit organizations exempt from federal and in many cases state premium taxes. It has been argued that without the community rating system this favored status is unjustified,[15] but the competitive advantage conferred by the exemption appears to be counterbalanced by restrictions on reserves that go with nonprofit status.[16]

More important advantages have flowed from the discounted rates Blue Cross plans were able to negotiate with participating hospitals. The ability to do so derived largely from their providing service benefits rather than the cash indemnity characteristic of commercial insurance. Carriers offering service benefits, including most Blue Cross plans and some Blue Shield plans, as well as Medicare and Medicaid, negotiate prior agreements with providers to pay specified rates. Blue Cross in many cases has been able to establish rate schedules based on actual costs, somewhat below the hospital's usual schedule of charges which allows for debt amortization, charity care, and overhead factors. Blue Shield has been less successful in this process of trying to persuade participating physicians to accept scheduled fees as payment in full.

Inconsistencies in the rates paid by various third parties and by individuals have been a much criticized consequence of this basic difference in approach. Government programs tend to pay lower rates, and the case is often made that this situation forces an indirect subsidy by the private sector of patients who are publicly financed. In some instances, private patients may pay as much as a 30 percent surcharge for hospital care. Uniform, cost-based rates, the argument continues, would require that subsidies be made explicit, an open public policy decision. There is support in the Carter administration for uniform rates of payment, but there is no reason to believe that a change would measurably affect the aggregate cost of care.

The service benefit has been a two-edged sword, like the community rating though to a lesser extent, placing Blue Cross at a competitive disadvantage vis-à-vis the commercial carriers. The commercial cash indemnity insurance appealed to employers and unions who wished insularity from controversy over the organization or adequacy of care.[17] It better suited the purposes of industry-wide bargaining for large and geographically dispersed beneficiaries because cash benefits permitted uniformity across areas with variable health care resources. Moreover, as the usual practice of the large carriers, cash indemnity health insurance could be purchased as part of a fuller package including other employee benefits. Over the years, increasing numbers of Blue Cross and Blue Shield plans have offered indemnity coverage, have given up local autonomy in favor of syndicates better able to serve a wider geographic area, and have generally yielded to the competitive pressures of the commercial carriers.

But 1965 brought a second turning point, possibly more important than the influence of World War II wage controls. The enactment of Medicare in that year brought the federal government into the health insurance system as a third large component. Though strictly speaking not an insurance program, Medicaid emerged that same year and contributed, with Medicare, to a massive infusion of federal funds into the health care system. Now a decade later, the two government financing programs have propelled the public share of national expenditures for personal health care to almost 40 percent,[18] and justify—some would say necessitate—the government's dominant voice in the articulation of health policy.

A chronology of the ebb and flow of the health insurance market, and even more the advent of the federal government as the heaviest investor of all, tends to obscure an essential point that bears repeating. If there is one unalterable truth about the financing of health care it is that whatever the structure or scheme, the public ultimately pays.[19] We sometimes forget that:

> *Americans have a very peculiar attitude toward government. To me, it is not the government who pays; the government receives it from us. Whether we say we are paying for health care out of pocket, by insurance, or by taxation, it still means we pay— through one of three different pockets. It is ridiculous to quarrel endlessly over which pocket is most burdened if I'm the last resort to fund the lot.*
>
> Theodore E. Chester

The financing of much of health insurance through the employment relationship conveys the oversimplified impression that the benefit is being bought by—or won from—the employer on the worker's behalf. In reality, the impression is only superficially accurate: health benefits are one part of the total compensation package and compete with other benefits or with wages for a finite amount of money. Far from being adversaries, management and labor have a joint and sometimes nearly equal stake in keeping costs in line. The Council on Wage and Price Stability identifies the common ground: "Health insurance premium expenses increase employer labor costs. Employers may strive to adjust by limiting further hiring, by pursuing other cost-reducing strategies, or by raising prices if market conditions allow. They may choose to, or have to, earn lower profits. In most cases, however, an indirect cost is imposed on the individual household through lower wages or higher prices."[20]

An Expanding Benefit Package

Reporting on a comprehensive survey of employee benefits, a 1974 Conference Board Publication offered the following overview:

> Employee benefits as we know them today issued from the marriage of employee beneficial associations and paternalism. Legitimatized by the courts and such institutions as insurance companies and banks, they have been propelled to their current importance by union pressure, and refined by consultants and corporate staff experts. They range in worth from $1 coffee breaks to billion-dollar trust funds. They form one of the most complex areas for government and corporate interaction, but also preserve such personal touches as a week off to get married or a widow's pension. They are based on essentially egalitarian concepts, such as actuarial tables and group purchasing power, yet they are used to mark status within and among companies. And, in some firms, they still separate the blue-collar and white-collar employee groups as if they were Indian castes. . . . In a way they are a hallmark of American big business.[1]

Health insurance comes in two basic forms: protection to maintain beneficiaries' or their dependents' incomes should their earning ability be cut off by death or disability; and coverage of medical expenses incurred as a result of illness or injury. The focus here is principally on the latter—health care plans designed to help workers and their dependents meet medical expenses.

Thus narrowed, the field remains bewilderingly complex. Over 1,500 health insurance carriers in the United States offer a multiplicity of plans and benefit packages (see box pp. 16–17), about 80 percent of which emanate from the employment relationship.[2] Current data on the extent of health insurance coverage through employee benefit plans seldom show the serious gaps in coverage that certainly exist. It is clear that there are wide variations in all kinds of employee benefits by industry, by region, by size of firm, and by level and status of the employee (office or nonoffice, permanent, part-time, on leave, striking, laid off, or retired as well as seniority with the firm).[3,4] The presence or absence of a union is another variable of consequence. Despite the influence unions have had on the scope of all employees' coverage, only about 25 percent of American workers are unionized, and fewer still belong to the benefits-rich, large industrial unions, such as those representing the auto, steel, rubber, aluminum, aerospace, and communications workers, the meat cutters, and others.

AN OVERVIEW OF HEALTH INSURANCE

Commercial insurance carriers consist of about 1,000 stock and mutual companies with the top twenty accounting for over 70 percent of the premium volume among this group. For them, health insurance is relatively new and usually a secondary line of insurance, but commercial carriers write over 50 percent of job-related hospital insurance and account for over half the nation's gross enrollment in health insurance generally.

Blue Cross and Blue Shield are nonprofit, tax-exempt health service prepayment plans for hospitalization (Blue Cross) and physicians' medical and surgical services (Blue Shield). Autonomous local plans are governed by boards of directors, required by law to include a majority of public representatives. In most states, they are regulated by a state insurance commission. There are sixty-nine Blue Cross and sixty-nine Blue Shield plans which are voluntarily affiliated nationally with the separate Blue Cross Association or Blue Shield Association. Customarily, though not necessarily sold together, Blue Cross and Blue Shield plans write about 40 to 45 percent of job-related insurance.

The government (federal and state) pays over one-third of total personal health care expenditures. The nationwide *Medicare* program (Title XVIII) insures people aged 65 or older and certain others and pays through a trust fund made up of payroll taxes and premiums from beneficiaries. Medicare is actually two programs, Part A for hospitalization and Part B for supplementary medical insurance. *Medicaid* (Title XIX) is not true insurance because it involves no premium payment by or for the beneficiary. It is a federally mandated and aided but state-administered program providing health care benefits for certain low income persons, some 25 million in 1975. *Workers' compensation* programs are state-run social insurance programs which provide income replacement and benefits covering some or all medical care costs resulting from job-related injury or illness.

Independent plans account for about 5 percent of hospital and 7 percent of medical and surgical coverage. They include (1) *Health Maintenance Organizations* (HMOs), which are organized delivery systems providing an agreed-upon set of basic and supplemental services to a voluntarily enrolled-population for a predetermined, fixed, periodic prepayment unrelated to the kind and amount of services used by the enrollee. HMOs come in two major types: the *prepaid group practice* in which physicians usually practice full-time at a central ambulatory care facility and earn a preestablished sum, perhaps supplemented by a bonus; and the *independent practice association,* in which physicians participate part-time in their own offices while maintaining their own independent practices. As of mid-1976, 175 prepaid health programs (HMOs) in the United States had just over 6 million subscribers. Of those 90 percent of the subscribers and 62 percent of the programs were of the prepaid group practice type. (2) *Employer-employee and union groups* cover about 6 million people or nearly 3 percent of the insured population. The size of the plans varies widely and a few large ones (for example, the United Mine Workers' of America Health and Retirement Funds, the National Association of Letter Carriers Health Benefits Plan; the National Postal Union Health Benefit Plan) account for most of that enrollment. Included here are roughly 3,000 "Taft-Hartley trusts" which are jointly administered by trustees representing both management and labor, and nearly 200 plans administered solely by workers or their representatives. The former tend to be multiemployer plans in industries, such as construction and transportation, characterized by large numbers of small firms.

Other channels for third-party financing of health care include employee benefit plans that are self-insured by the employer; and certain elements of automobile, homeowners, and accident insurance.

Sources:

Blue Cross Association and Blue Shield Association: *1977 Fact Book* (Chicago: Blue Cross Association and Blue Shield Association, 1977).

Executive Office of the President, Council on Wage and Price Stability: *The Complex Puzzle of Rising Health Care Costs: Can the Private Sector Fit it Together?* (Washington, D.C.: USGPO no. 053–003–0025508, December 1976).

Health Insurance Institute: *Source Book of Health Insurance Data, 1976–77* (New York: Health Insurance Institute, 1977).

Krizay, John, and Andrew Wilson: *The Patient As Consumer* (Lexington, Mass.: Lexington Books, 1974).

Price, Daniel N. "Private Health Insurance Plans: Type of Administration and Insurer in 1974," *Social Security Bulletin,* March 1977, pp. 13–42.

Skolnik, Alfred M. "Twenty-Five Years of Employee Benefit Plans," *Social Security Bulletin,* September 1976, pp. 3–21.

Strumpf, George B: "Health Maintenance Organizations, 1971 to 1976: Issues and Answers," paper presented at 104th annual meeting of the American Public Health Association, Miami Beach, Fla., October 19, 1976.

Subcommittee on Health and the Environment, Committee on Interstate and Foreign Commerce, U.S. House of Representatives: *A Discursive Dictionary of Health Care* (Washington, D.C.: USGPO no. 052–070–03199–9, 1976).

Weeks, David A.: *National Health Insurance and Corporate Benefit Plans: An Interim Report* (New York: Conference Board, 1975).

Statistics on health insurance are available from private and public sources. The Health Insurance Institute publishes an annual compilation of health insurance data, largely from the perspective of the insurance industry for which the institute speaks. Along with data on the extent and scope of coverage, the 1976–77 edition includes a brief narrative description of the history of health insurance and efforts by insurers to help contain costs. The United States Chamber of Commerce produces a biennial report on employee benefits which aggregates old age, survivors, disability, and health insurance data, making it difficult to draw conclusions about health benefits alone. Reports from the Office of Research and Statistics of the Social Security Administration and from the Bureau of Labor Statistics appear periodically in the *Social Security Bulletin* and elsewhere. These are informative, as was the Conference Board's 1974 report. Since 1950 the Social Security Administration has collected data and prepared annual reports on coverage, contributions, and benefits under employee benefit plans. Detailed information on health care benefits is therefore available but is largely beyond the scope of this monograph.

Recent trends in coverage are relevant, however, especially where they illuminate industry's perspective on rising health care costs. Helpful in this regard is a survey of twenty-five years of employee benefit plans, published in the September 1976 *Social Security Bulletin*. The survey shows that collective bargaining pressures during the 1950s caused rapid growth in the proportion of the labor force covered by all employee benefits during that decade. In 1950 half the wage and salary labor force was covered by some health insurance; by 1960, two-thirds. The 1960s brought a leveling off of the trend to expand coverage (to 71 percent of the work force by 1970 and slightly lower, proportionately, by 1974), with a concurrent liberalization of benefits for those already covered. There has been a shift, more pronounced during the 1960s than the 1970s, toward elimination of employee contributions for coverage, first of hospitalization and then of medical and surgical care, and a progressive raising of the ceiling on coverage in order to better protect against catastrophic expenses. A 1959 steelworkers' strike led the way for noncontributory coverage for employees' health care benefits and the automobile industry followed the lead in 1961. By 1972 employers nationwide were paying about half the total premium cost; by 1975 it was two-thirds of the total, with about 40 percent of employers paying 100 percent of the premium for their employees' health care benefits.[5]

Finally, the last decade has seen a significant broadening of the base of coverage to include new types of services, notably care provided in nonhospital settings. Again, collectively bargained plans provide the principal stimulus—for prepaid dental care, negotiated between 1971 and 1974 by the auto workers, steelworkers, and at least four other large industrial unions; for out-of-hospital prescription drugs, first negotiated in 1967 by the auto workers; and probably in the near future, for vision care benefits, foreshadowed by their inclusion in the auto workers' 1976 negotiated package.[6] Nursing home care constitutes another rapidly expanding benefit.[7]

At first glance, the long-range trend looks undeniably healthy, with expanding then deepening coverage, wider limits on out-of-pocket liability, and a growing willingness on the part of employers to shoulder the bulk of the financial burden—progress that seems to overshadow the deceleration in the proportion of workers covered. On closer scrutiny, however, signs of pathology emerge. During the last 15 years of the Social Security Administration's 25-year retrospective review, the substantial dollar increases observed in employee and employer contributions "to a large extent merely reflected rising hospital costs." In fact, the report states, "the difficulties encountered by many plans in keeping their cash allowances up to date has led to a shift away from cash indemnity to full service benefits, which have the advantage of providing automatic protection against rising costs."[8]

It is limited protection indeed, leading the next year to higher premiums, absorbed by employer, employee, or both. The expanded coverage, to some extent, is a smokescreen obscuring the progressive erosion in the dollar value of the benefit package had it remained unchanged. Unions have responded to the devaluation of their health benefits by trying first to negotiate larger packages to offset health care cost inflation and, failing that, to bargain for low-cost expansions in the package in an attempt to justify higher premiums, for example, higher maxima on days of hospitalization covered or coverage of illnesses such as drug addiction and alcoholism—"important but not costly changes that help explain rises in premium rates to the union membership."[9]

In the end, as the Council on Wage and Price Stability observes, there is no denying the relationship of these trends to the total wage package. "Between 1965 and 1973, annual contributions to employee health benefit plans (including both employer and employee shares) jumped 164 percent from $7.5 billion to $19.8 billion. Health benefits are thus becoming an ever larger portion of total compensation costs. Both union and management leaders have expressed concern over further cost increases in the health benefit component of labor compensation and their potential impact upon prices, wages, and profits."[10] Organized labor's appreciation of the potential threat to wages and other benefits contained in rising health care costs is said to account in large measure for its long-standing support of mandatory national health insurance financed by means other than premiums—as a way of removing health care from the bargaining table.

Some Causes and Effects of Rising Costs

Economists tend to disagree on the relative importance of various factors contributing to inflation in health care costs: "Long lists of explanations have been presented to account for persistently high rates of increases in health expenditures. . . . It is fair to say that there is still no consensus among economists, even when they look at the same data, on the reasons. . . . In these circumstances, it is not surprising that the policy proposals offered to remedy the escalation of expenditures differ a great deal."[1]

Without becoming embroiled in the subtleties of the economists' debate, it seems safe to generalize that the financing system for health services is both cause and effect of rising health care costs, driving them upward in a vicious circle. Since private industry, as payer for care, has long been intimately involved in the financing of health services, the relationship of the financing system to the cost of care is relevant as a backdrop against which to see industry's role in controlling costs:

> *As medical care costs have risen, the pressure has come on indus-try to expand the medical care coverage for its employees—both the percentage of costs covered and the scope of services. A prime reason for the pressure is that if you guys pay the bill for my premium you don't have to pay income tax on my income and I don't have to pay income tax on my income, and that's a good deal.*

Judith R. Lave

Fringe benefits are deductible as corporate business expenses and are not taxable as part of the employee's individual income. "This creates a tax incentive for employees to bargain for generous employer-provided health benefits: the employer dollar spent for health insurance buys more coverage than would the same dollar paid as a wage, taxed, and the balance spent by the employee for health insurance."[2] As a result, there has been a discernable trend toward the employer's assuming a growing proportion of the cost of health insurance. In the 80 percent of group insurance plans that are employment-related, the employer pays, on the average, 67 percent of the total premium. Forty-one percent of these plans are noncontributory, that is, the employer pays the full premium.[3]

Some researchers believe that the tax advantage has been a major deter-minant of insurance coverage, promoting "too much of the wrong kind of health protection"—shallow, "first-dollar" coverage and inadequate insurance against unpredictable, catastrophic costs.[4] In emphasizing hospital-based, high-technology care, it is argued, and by removing cost as a relevant consider-ation in the patient's decision to seek care and the physician's decision to order it, insurance plans have produced incentives that have elevated demand for these expensive services. For example, Martin Feldstein observes, in 1950 the average cost per day of hospitalization was $16; by 1974, $125. Meanwhile, the average share of the bill financed through public and private insurance increased from 37 to 77 percent. The net cost to the average patient was $10 and $28.50 respectively, or, corrected for inflation, $10 and $13. Because individu-als with private coverage are covered for 79 percent of their hospital bills, on average, an extra $10 of expensive care costs the consumer only $2 out of pocket.[5]

The paradoxical concept that insurance creates excessive demand for health services is now widely held. The rationale for health insurance, of course, is to spread the risk across a group of beneficiaries and thus, in effect, to remove financial barriers to care for the individuals in the group with the greatest need. Government financing programs—Medicare and Medicaid espe-cially—are deliberately designed to enlarge access to health care for groups with unmet needs. Evidence that objective need might *not* be the dominant force in health care began to surface during the late 1950s. Members of prepaid group practices were using substantially fewer hospital days than comparable groups of subscribers to conventional insurance plans. In 1959, Milton Roemer advanced the theory that supply in the hospital sector creates its own demand. Needed or not, he observed, existing hospital beds tend to be filled and paid for.[6] Subsequently elaborated and expanded to encompass health services generally, the theory derives from the intuition that providers more than patients dictate the nature and extent of the health services that are consumed. The physician, as the expert, makes or guides the decision. The patient, often under stress at the time the decision must be made, tends not to factor in cost as a relevant consideration, especially because the third-party payment masks its financial impact. Widespread third-party payment in a sense releases providers and consumers from any obligation to concern themselves with costs:

> *The world was very simple in the days before insurance came into full flower. There was not only a patient–physician relationship, a professional relationship, there was also an economic relationship. The physician knew the patient's family and financial circumstances and was mindful in making a medical decision of its economic consequences for the patient.*
>
> John J. Boardman, Jr.

Insurance coverage for the consequences of those medical decisions has given rise to a different kind of simple rule: the Medical Uncertainty Principle. Because "medicine is only partially and imperfectly related to health," Aaron Wildavsky argues, "doctor and patient both are uncertain as to what is wrong or what to do about it. . . . The Medical Uncertainty Principle states that there is always one more thing that might be done—another consultation, a new drug, a different treatment. Uncertainty is resolved by doing more: the patient asks for more, the doctor orders more. The patient's simple rule for resolving uncertainty is to seek care up to the level of his insurance."[7] Little is to be gained by trying to sort out the blame. Almost no group is without some responsibility in the complex calculus of social, economic, technological, and political forces, the professional prerogatives, and the public expectations underlying the present character of the health care delivery system:

> *The primary concern of the consumer is a cure. It's not even mysticism regarding medicine, simply that this is a highly technological society. There's no time to fool around when one goes to the doctor; I want a pill, a prescription, a procedure, and when I leave your office, I want to be better in 24 hours; don't bother me with details. So, while we complain about the provider in his role as the agent for the consumer, that consumer comes in here with some expectations to buy a way to better health.*
>
> Spencer C. Johnson

More important than assigning blame is deciding what can be done. And it is increasingly evident that if private industry has been part of the problem, it can certainly be part of the solution. Perhaps, the Council on Wage and Price Stability suggests, even the key to the solution. "Cost control incentives proposed by the private sector—that is, by industry and labor—promise to be more effective than those that have been imposed by the multitude of government agencies which have attempted to tackle the problem."[8]

Approaches to Cost Containment

Most of the innovations being tried by private industry in its role as payer for health care originate in attempts to bring premiums under control. Independently of the motives from which they spring, however, some approaches have the wider potential of improving the external delivery system. As industry's sophistication in health services grows, this secondary societal effect is now being consciously sought in increasing numbers of instances:

> Historically, employers have employed relatively few people in health benefits administration; there has been rather unquestioning acceptance of the insurance carrier and medical professional; and data upon which policy decisions should be made was minimal. Today, all this is changing. More people are being hired to work in health benefits—and they are frequently young professionals with more knowledge of health issues than of the company's products. Self-insurance has proven financially attractive to many and also has increased the incentive for direct intervention in the local health scene. Data is rapidly being accumulated resulting in an employer-consumer who can meet the provider on equal terms.[1]

The role of payer for care is probably the best established of industry's three major roles in health care, and it is here that industry has developed the greatest array of creative cost control strategies. Indeed, the diversity of approaches can be confusing, in the absence of a conceptual matrix within which to sort and assess them. A simplified scheme has been suggested by the assistant vice president for health care systems at Employers Insurance of Wausau:

> *Although many things affect the cost of health care, there are really only three that determine the insurance premium: the fee for administration, the utilization of services, and the charge for those services. While it is possible to attack the administrative side of things and to institute very sophisticated management information programs, it is essential to attack all three to be effective. Utilization is controlled in part by medical providers and consumers but is influenced by the benefit package. Fees and charges of all providers can be negotiated in advance.*
>
> Jacob J. Spies

The cost containment strategies initiated by industry as payer are grouped here in those three categories. As a principal orientation, each one can be said to address either: the costs of administering a benefit package; the utilization of services financed by that package; or the charges for the services used (see figure 5). The objectives and rationale behind each approach are described here briefly, and major unresolved issues identified. Some illustrations are provided; many more can be found in the Council on Wage and Price Stability's compendium. Our purpose here is not to probe deeply into the details of particular cost containment strategies—especially since specific information is available elsewhere—but rather to meld the available information on industry's activities with other information from the medical care literature and so to lay the substratum for future volumes in the Springer Series.

Many of the approaches included here are based not on empirical evidence of effectiveness but on assumptions derived from beliefs or observations about the reasons for current problems. That is, they tend to be reactive. For example, if cost problems are thought to stem from retrospective cost-based reimbursement of hospitals, from insurance coverage of hospitalization to the exclusion of less costly alternatives, or from too much surgery, then solutions are sought, respectively, in prospective reimbursement, coverage of outpatient care, and second opinion surgery. The logic can be unassailable, but lacking previous experience, there are practical problems in implementation, not the least of which are unintended side effects. Seldom have the results of the strategies been evaluated systematically. These defects are endemic to public sector approaches as well, and can, for the most part, be attributed to rapidly unfolding change. Many will doubtless yield to time and further refinement.

Addressing Administrative Costs

To achieve more efficient financing of a given benefit package, industry is adopting numerous mechanisms for reviewing and controlling claims, computerizing processes and reducing paperwork, verifying hospital admissions and lengths of stay, ascertaining whether services billed were really performed, auditing bills and the extent to which they are covered under the employee benefit agreement, and coordinating benefits. Claims review is often triggered automatically when the bill reaches a preestablished threshold. A purely administrative mechanism, claims review is normally retrospective; concurrent or prospective review seeks to intervene and affect inappropriate utilization.

As a group, these administrative refinements emanate from a building perception that laxity has existed and is becoming intolerably expensive. For example, Standard Oil of California estimates that mere coordination of benefits (COB)—a procedure to minimize the cost of duplicate claims under overlapping policies even if underwritten by different carriers—saved the corporation $18.6 million in 1973, $22.6 million in 1974, and $32 million in 1975.[2]

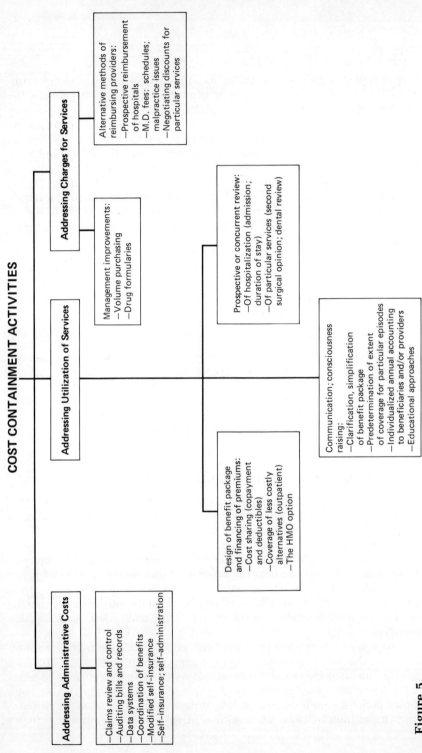

COST CONTAINMENT ACTIVITIES

Addressing Administrative Costs

—Claims review and control
—Auditing bills and records
—Data systems
—Coordination of benefits
—Modified self-insurance
—Self-insurance; self-administration

Addressing Utilization of Services

Design of benefit package
and financing of premiums:
—Cost sharing (copayment
and deductibles)
—Coverage of less costly
alternatives (outpatient)
—The HMO option

Communication; consciousness
raising:
—Clarification, simplification
of benefit package
—Predetermination of extent
of coverage for particular episodes
—Individualized annual accounting
to beneficiaries and/or providers
—Educational approaches

Prospective or concurrent review:
—Of hospitalization (admission;
duration of stay)
—Of particular services (second
surgical opinion; dental review)

Addressing Charges for Services

Management improvements:
—Volume purchasing
—Drug formularies

Alternative methods of
reimbursing providers:
—Prospective reimbursement
of hospitals
—M.D. fees: schedules;
malpractice issues
—Negotiating discounts for
particular services

Figure 5.

Equitable Life estimated in 1976 that the aggregate COB savings possible for all third-party payers is close to $1 billion per year.[2]

Overall, the effect of admistrative improvements is largely limited to the individual company—indeed to a single budget item. One broader implication may be the generation of data—a requisite not only of streamlined administration but of most other cost control initiatives as well. "As purchasers of health benefits, corporations have been unable to determine whether or not they and their employees are getting the best value for the dollar. Valid and meaninful data are essential if any measurement of the services is even to be attempted."[3] With adequate data systems in place, multistate corporations and unions are well situated to identify hitherto unrecognized anomalies in the delivery and costs of health services.

Another possible broader-range implication relates to the issue, now much in the public eye, of fraud and abuse by providers of health care. Claims review involves, in part, a verification that the procedures billed for were really provided. This suggests to Goldbeck of the Washington Business Group on Health that industry will need to be willing to press charges when evidence of fraud is uncovered, and to monitor fraud and abuse as the federal government is beginning to do in its Medicare and Medicaid programs.[4] "Otherwise there is no reason to assume that the private sector won't be subjected to 'spillover fraud' in close proportion to the degree of success the government has in reducing fraud in its own programs." Enlisting the employee-patient in the review of claims, Goldbeck argues, can be of great assistance in detecting and preventing fraud and can also serve useful educational functions.[5]

Beyond these specific refinements, the ultimate step large employers and employee groups are taking toward administrative control of premium costs is to "self-insure" for health care and eliminate the middleman. Self-insurance "is a misnomer meaning simply that the company does not insure for health care."[6] In testimony to the Council on Wage and Price Stability, the Washington Business Group on Health reported that eight of ninty-three companies surveyed were self-insured, nineteen partially so, and eighteen more planning to move to self-insurance.[6]

Because of experience rating, state premium taxes, and the insurance companies' practice of retaining a portion of the premium as a reserve, it is sometimes argued that most large purchasers of health insurance ought to be self-insured.

> I'm convinced that very few companies with 500 or more employees should be using conventional insurance as it has existed for decades with full reserves held by the insurance company. It's a foolhardy arrangement unless there are other priorities taking precedence over the cost of the benefit package. Conventionally insured programs are just not cost-efficient. You must start with the assumption that companies of this size are self-insured right now. Insurance carriers will not call it that and may argue that they are offering important protection, but it is protection against one-year cash flow problems, not against adverse experience. Most health

care insurance plans are not insurance at all. My surprise is that
more companies have not moved to adopting various degrees of
self-insurance.

Michael B. Jones

The intermediate steps that Jones suggests large purchases can take on the way to full self-insurance and self-administration include such procedures as negotiating with the carriers over commissions and administrative charges, assuming some of the risk for adverse fluctuations in claims, reducing or eliminating the reserves that the insurance companies carry (which, in conventional arrangements, can equal 35 to 45 percent of paid claims in a year), eliminating dividends (that is, year-end returns to the company from the insurance carrier), and establishing various alternative funding mechanisms such as interim accounting which allows for adjustment of the reserve at various points throughout the year.

Self-insurance approaches go. back at least to the 1950s. Cost advantages flow from administrative savings, interest on reserve credit, and elimination of state premium taxes, which in most states private insurance carriers have to pay but self-insuring employers need not. Other advantages have been claimed as well:

Deere and Company, which has 50,000 employees, went to self-
administration about seven years ago and has considerable experi-
ence. The break-even point depends on many factors: the number
of employees, where they are concentrated, and the complexity
and comprehensiveness of the benefit package. Our experience.
shows that we are administering our own plan at a rate appreciably
less than the best rate we could obtain from an insurance company,
and that does not take into account the interest on reserve credit
and the state premium taxes. There are other advantages that we
think we obtain as well—a more coordinated approach and better
employee understanding. The union likes the plan.

Kevin Stokeld

Self-insurance gives the large purchaser direct control over provider reimbursement and the collection of data, increasing the leverage that can be applied against the delivery system or individual components thereof. That leverage increases with the proportion of a given provider's or vendor's business accounted for by members of the group represented by the self-insuring purchaser. When 40 percent of a clinic's patients are beneficiaries of the United Mines Workers' Health and Retirement Fund, for instance, the administrator of that clinic will probably be quite receptive to suggestions from spokesmen for the Fund. For Goodyear Tire & Rubber in Akron, Ohio, 20 years of self-insurance has generated data and control which the company has recently been able to parlay into substantial legitimacy and influence in the community health planning process,[7] as discussed more fully in chapter 4.

Self-insurance may also have a synergistic effect with other cost containment programs. For example, a second surgical opinion program may have higher chances of success if combined with self-insurance so that the employee benefit manager has timely access to information on members scheduled for surgery.[8]

Obliquely, self-insurance raises a complex and controversial issue: the potential role of the insurance companies in controlling health care costs. Researchers who have looked at the question are divided in their conclusions[9,10] and the myriad national health insurance proposals before Congress reflect this diversity of opinion. Large companies and large groups may do better by "going self-insured," but they are sometimes reluctant to do so for fear of rocking the boat of the insurance industry. And if in moving to self-insurance they take the next logical step and begin using their leverage to negotiate discounted rates, they may leave the smaller groups and individuals to fend for themselves. Moreover, if self-insurance becomes widespread, state governments will no doubt find ways to recover the tax revenue lost in health insurance premium taxes, and will thus remove some of the financial advantage now realizable through self-insurance.

In summary, the strategies aimed at administrative costs are relatively straightforward. Their time horizon is short. Their impact is felt quickly but is limited in scope because it does not address the fundamental causes of rising health care costs:

> *The primary thing is that the insurance premium, really, is a function of health care costs, and not the other way around. As we talk about these kinds of negotiations with the insurance companies, we have to remember that there are deeper problems here that we should be getting through to.*
>
> Jacob J. Spies

Addressing Utilization of Services

The utilization of medical services is one of those critical "deeper problems"—and one to which industry in its role as purchaser of care may have unusual access. Cost containment approaches addressing appropriate use take the form of modifications to the benefit package to alter the incentives it produces, and various prospective review programs designed to forestall inappropriate use of hospitalization and other medical services. Most of the programs in this category have a strong educational thrust: whether stated or implicit, there is usually an underlying goal of heightening the consciousness of beneficiaries concerning prudent and effective use of the medical care system, and, to a lesser extent, that of providers concerning the need to moderate costs.

Ideally, one would like this to be a two-way communication, with employees—whether unionized or not—actively participating in decisions about the scope of health benefits and the trade-offs implied in the choice of one package over another. It is not uncommon for companies to conduct surveys to gauge employee opinion of their benefits and to factor this information into the decisions that are made. But it appears that more work could be done to find effective ways of enlisting real employee participation in the process of designing the benefit package.

Benefit Package and Premium Financing

Changing the benefit package—with varying degrees of subtlety and sophistication—is in some form or another a nearly universal strategy among large-scale payers for medical insurance. In principle, it is corrective: it seeks to replace the faulty incentives that are blamed for cost escalation with a benefit package that promotes less costly alternatives—usually meaning care requiring fewer hospital days or avoiding the hospital altogether. Justified on grounds that more utilization of medical care is often not "better" and can indeed be "worse" for the patient than is less care, the most obvious benefit modification—consumer cost-sharing—is introduced through the vehicle of coinsurance and deductibles.

Cost-sharing is viewed as a means of reintroducing an element of personal financial responsibility for health care and hence of discouraging excess utilization. Under coinsurance, the insured shares costs with the insurer according to a fixed ratio (say, 20:80 or 40:60 with the carrier normally assuming the larger portion, but sometimes 50:50) and usually only up to a maximum out-of-pocket cost. Deductibles refer to the amount of covered expenses that must be borne by the beneficiary before the insurer begins to pay the benefits. The cost-sharing provision in both cases is applied to a specific benefit: hospitalization, physicians' services, dental or vision care, or whatever.

Coinsurance and deductibles are frequently found in major medical insurance policies, the fastest growing type of policy since its introduction in 1951 in response to a demand for protection against large, unpredictable expenses. Deductibles presume that the insured can budget for routine medical expenses and are thus a logical corollary to the concept of insurance against major episodes of illness.

Collectively bargained plans have led the movement away from cost-sharing, and unions are predictably opposed to retrenchment on this point, as evidenced by testimony to the Council on Wage and Price Stability by the Amalgamated Clothing and Textile Workers: "Cost controls that put the burden on the patient to limit their use of health services such as copayments, deductibles, time limits, dollar limits, and other artificial means of control can only result in some people not getting the medical care they need because they can't afford it. These kinds of controls make a mockery of the concept of preventive medicine and early treatment and detection of disease."[11]

As the testimony suggests, the inequity of erecting barriers to appropriate use of health services by the poor and needy is the principal argument adduced by opponents of cost-sharing. A study of cost-sharing under public health insurance in Canada did find that the burden fell disproportionately on lower-income beneficiaries.[12] A California study found that the introduction of coinsurance in a prepaid plan diminished the plan's ability to enroll lower-income subscribers.[13,14] Fine tuning of the coinsurance and deductible provisions (for example, scaling them to income) may be a way to mitigate, but probably not obviate, problems of equal access to needed care. Cost-sharing is expensive to administer if it is finely tuned but risks being inequitable if it is not.

One economist argues that practical difficulties (union opposition and willingness on the part of some consumers to buy supplementary insurance filling the gaps left by coinsurance and deductibles) would probably thwart wide-scale implementation of cost-sharing measures, and that, furthermore, "copayment may involve greater costs than benefits and is not a good solution."[15] The impact of coinsurance on utilization of medical services is difficult to isolate definitively. The "experiment" is almost always "contaminated" by some other modifications to the benefit package, usually made in an effort to "soften the blow" of a newly instituted cost sharing provision.[16]

The June 1977 decision by the United Mine Workers of America Health and Retirement Funds to institute significant cost-sharing may lead to some new insights on the effects on utilization of services. Faced with a shortfall in the funds, the trustees instituted 60:40 coinsurance, with the patient paying 40 percent for all physicians' fees (inpatient and outpatient) and a $250 deductible for hospital service charges, with a $500 annual ceiling on a family's out-of-pocket obligation. Equipped with a new data system, the administrators of the funds intend to study the results systematically.[17]

Opposition and ambiguity notwithstanding, cost-sharing seems to be on the increase. In testimony before the Council on Wage and Price Stability and in written submissions to the Washington Business Group on Health, numerous corporate spokesmen described actions or plans to increase coinsurance and deductibles, if not on currently available benefits, then on new ones to be offered in the future. At the Cornell Conference for Business Executives, cost-sharing was much on participants' minds. The following exchange was typical:

Audience comment: Three years ago, our company was paying one-third of the premium. Then we went to one-half, and last year to two-thirds. What we have been doing is absorbing the increasing cost of health care while the employee contribution remains level. But now we're in a situation where to continue this policy we would have to pay about seven-eighths of the costs. Is it possible to say to the employees that they will have to absorb perhaps a 10 percent increase? In your experience, would they accept that?

Michael B. Jones: Yes, it is a problem. How do you approach the employees and what do you tell them? And where is their threshold of pain? In some corporations you couldn't get by with much at all. But it's a judgment factor and I don't think there's any magic formula. A couple of my clients who had a noncontributory plan because they moved with the trend five to ten years ago, are now starting to charge employees a percentage. When they do that it's with very careful communication, believe me, and not without some employee resentment. But typically, people are understanding.

Thomas E. Burns: It's difficult to do. What develops is a sense of entitlement on the part of the employees, and in the history of negotiations, very few of those benefits are taken away once they are given.

In much of the discussion by proponents of cost-sharing, there is a tentative tone that conveys uncertainty about potential impact on costs, and a sense that the *educational* objective may be paramount.

I've certainly seen a lot of companies passing on the costs of a plan to employees recently. Some employers figure that this is a way to increase employees' sensitivity to health care costs. When they get a medical cost increase they pass some of it on to their employees, just so that the employees are aware of what's happening.
Michael B. Jones

Coverage of cost-reducing alternatives flips the cost-sharing coin. Rather than discourage undesired use of facilities or services, it is a mechanism to encourage use of facilities and services thought to be at least as appropriate medically and probably less expensive. Among the alternatives now being covered by liberalized benefits, some are designed to reduce hospitalization: preadmission testing, ambulatory care and outpatient surgery, home health care, and care in skilled nursing facilities others are intended to promote care viewed as prophylactic or preventive: dentistry, vision care, and mental health benefits. And at least one addresses the manpower pool: coverage of services rendered by qualified medical auxiliaries and paraprofessionals.

The rationale for restructuring the benefit package away from hospitalization is self-evident: the 1975 increase in hospital service charges was both the largest component of health care inflation (13 percent) and the most important because expenditures for hospital care constitute almost 40 percent of all health spending.[18] But health insurance traditionally shied away from these "less-medical" services, for fear the demand for them would be endless and overutilization a constant problem. Overuse of these outpatient "alternatives" is still a valid concern; adequate evidence is simply not in yet.

Another apparently cost-reducing option is the HMO. Well before the federal government enacted the Health Maintenance Organization Act of 1973, segments of private industry were offering membership in a prepaid plan as an option under employee health insurance, and some firms and unions were deeply involved in the development of prepaid plans. The federal statute, ostensibly seeking to give HMOs a boost, mandated employer provision of a dual option under certain circumstances for federally qualified HMOs, but set such unrealistic criteria for qualification as to hobble the HMO movement.[18] The mandatory dual option clause has been controversial and relatively inef-

fectual. Removal of informational entry barriers to HMO membership is necessary since a concerted educational effort may be needed before a prepaid plan
will effectively penetrate a new market. An enthusiastic employer can assist in
the educational process, but a reluctant one can satisfy the letter of the dual
option requirement while stimulating very little employee interest in the plan.

Some of the reasons for the slow growth of HMOs are discussed in
chapter 3, where readers unfamiliar with prepaid health programs will find
definitions and underlying concepts. The discussion here is limited to the role
of HMOs as a benefit modification.

Traditionally, the addition of an HMO option under the benefit plan
derived from philosophical rather than strictly cost-saving motivations—a
statement in favor of the beneficiary's freedom to choose and an endorsement of
the long-range potential of HMOs to reduce overutilization and perhaps
thereby to modulate costs. Employees who opt for the HMO generally receive a
more comprehensive range of medical benefits for a prepaid annual fee, originally but now progressively less often, entailing a slightly higher insurance
premium:

> The cost of the HMO plan is already lower than the conventional
> package in many communities and I predict this trend will con-
> tinue. This for two reasons: the slope of cost increases on the HMO
> side is slower than for the rest of the system, and benefits are
> expanding on the entire health insurance package so that the basic
> benefit package that these two options offer is coming closer and
> closer together.
>
> Paul M. Ellwood, Jr.

Usually, the employee electing HMO membership has been responsible
for paying the incremental cost of that coverage. Now that HMOs are beginning
to cost less than traditional coverage a dilemma arises:

> You'll be faced with a tough set of decisions as the prices of these
> two packages begin to pass each other. And I hope that industry's
> way of coping with it will not be to increase the scope of the
> benefits on the HMO side—by offering prepaid dental and the
> like—in order to equalize the costs. Because that will just drive up
> the costs of both sides. Better to equalize the costs by cutting
> benefits on the more costly side.
>
> Paul M. Ellwood, Jr.

It seems only fair that HMO subscribers, especially those who have been
paying a little more each month to belong to an HMO, should pay a little less
when the HMO premium falls below the cost of conventional coverage. Moreover, it may be important to allow the cost differential to show, especially since
an original objective of the HMO movement was to stimulate competition
among alternative delivery systems.

If additions to services and additions to premiums were closely related in the view of subscribers and potential subscribers, then they would have a way of deciding, in small enough groups to have an impact, what services they want included at what incremental cost. We need competing groups and differential premiums to reflect differences in services. And I would argue that, at the moment, with no cost differential, fee-for-service, private physician practice is probably the preferred souce of care.

Judith R. Lave

Many corporations and unions have now opened up an HMO option, but enrollment has often fallen short of expectations. General Motors' experience is not atypical:

General Motors has been involved in at least one or two HMOs for almost twenty-five years. Our experience is basically good and we support the concept. But there are great variations from area to area and from plan to plan in a number of things: the financial support the plan needs to get under way, and the quality of the medical staff, and the ability to retain good staff. HMOs have not spread because there are not enough people who know how to do the job, for one thing, and for a second, employees are very suspicious of the concept in many areas. Although about 60 percent of our people in the San Francisco area are HMO members, and about 35 percent in southern California and about 20 percent in Rochester, the story is different in other parts of the country. We recently held enrollments in three new areas, Cincinnati, Indianapolis, and Kansas City, and made special efforts to help employees understand the group practice arrangements. Despite our efforts, less than 1 percent of eligible employees enrolled and very few people were sufficiently interested to go and look at the facilities. There's a great reluctance on the part of individuals to give up the freedom they have with the present system.

Victor M. Zink

We at General Electric have had very similar experiences, that is very low participation, even in recent enrollments where our people worked with the HMO on the enrollment drive. We find that 1 percent or fewer employees opt for the HMO.

C. Stephen Tsorvas

In some parts of the country, by contrast, HMOs have done very well in enlisting employee enrollment. Minneapolis–St. Paul has seven operating HMOs, with, as of April 1, 1977, some 160,000 enrolled members. Most of those members, according to David F. McIntyre, manager of employee benefits for General Mills, "are covered under a group contract through the employment relationship:"

Now with seven HMOs vying for new members, there is an element of competition in the health delivery system. We are seeing compe-

tition in marketing, in services offered, and perhaps most importantly, in the cost of the particular benefit packages offered. From an employee benefits manager's standpoint and from that of the company, this makes for a much improved situation during a period of generally rising health care costs.

David F. McIntyre

The HMO movement may be regaining some of its lost momentum and, as new HMOs work to build up membership, they will certainly turn to industry for quick access to potentially large markets. Turning both to labor:

There is no question that Kaiser-Permanente's move to southern California was stimulated by the fact that the retail clerks and the longshoremen could deliver 30,000 people on April 1, 1951. Prior to the passage of the HMO Act, labor was a prime mover on Kaiser's behalf in many cases. UAW members went into our programs in California without our having a formal contractual relationship with Ford Motor Company or GM. The same is true of the Taft-Hartley trusts.

John J. Boardman, Jr.

and to management:

I can't see how we are going to begin restoring a market in health services without the business sector pushing it.

Paul M. Ellwood, Jr.

HMOs have ardent supporters and an established track record. In 1976 HMOs nationally increased their rates only 19 percent, while many third-party payers introduced rate hikes of 30 to 40 percent.[19] But legitimate questions are raised about whether HMOs can develop fast enough to meet a cost problem that is immediate:

Kaiser-Permanente has been in business since 1948. By now it has 3 million subscribers and the number is growing by 9 percent a year. Compounded, on a base of the 6 million people now served by HMOs, it's going to take 8 years to have 12 million members. With twice as many HMOs, 8 years to cover 24 million. And in 8 years the population will have grown, at present rates, by 12 million people. So the most optimistic estimates of how many people in this country HMOs will cover is way below what would be needed to restructure the system in a reasonable length of time. And we only have a reasonable length of time to come to grips with the problems that we are facing: health care cost escalation threatens to destroy the whole system.

Kenneth A. Platt

Platt's alternative is to place controls on the existing system through programs such as concurrent peer review of the quality and appropriateness of care.

Prospective and Concurrent Utilization Review

Conceptually, the chief distinction between retrospective claims review and both prospective and concurrent utilization review is a matter of timing. Prospective review programs include preadmission screening for hospitalization for certain specified procedures, second opinion programs prior to elective surgery, or prior to dental procedures and the like. Concurrent utilization review usually refers to in-hospital programs where a nurse or some other health professional certifies the appropriateness of a hospital admission and monitors the length of stay, based on established criteria taking account of the patient's age, sex, and diagnosis. These programs typically have a multilevel mechanism through which the attending physician can appeal the program's ruling to other physicians in the hospital and then to regional and state physician committees. In theory, the conduct of the review while a decision is being made to render a medical service allows the time to intervene and prevent an inappropriate choice. The distinction may be more theoretical than real, follow-up of findings can be a problem, and evidence to date suggests that savings achieved by quality assurance programs probably "come from administrative reviews of patient eligibility for insurance coverage, the range of reimbursable benefits, or the amount of reimbursement claimed ... savings which would be realized under most claims review systems and generally are unrelated to considerations of either quality or appropriateness of care."[20]

Because quality judgments are implicit in an assessment of the appropriateness of a medical order, utilization review typically goes hand in glove with "quality assurance" programs whose stated goal is to assure high quality medical care at a reasonable cost. These are complex and various, with considerable range as to, for example, the timing, depth, and frequency of review. Their background and context, along with salient issues they raise, have been well explored elsewhere and need only be sketched here in broadest outline.

Peer review of medical care has become the nearly exclusive domain of physician-dominated professional standards review organizations (PSROs), created as part of the 1972 amendments to the Social Security Act (P.L. 92-603). The purpose of the PSRO program is to assure that medical services financed through three government programs, Medicare, Medicaid, and Child Health and Crippled Childrens' Services, are medically necessary, in accord with professionally recognized standards, and appropriately provided in the most economical setting. Independently of the medical facilities they evaluate, PSROs develop and use local standards of appropriate hospital admission, length of stay, and course of treatment, and are responsible for reviewing care either directly or by monitoring the performance of a facility's medical staff utilization review committee to whom the PSRO can delegate the review. PSROs are now operating in at least 120 of the 203 areas into which the program has carved the country. As they get under way, PSROs will oversee, be accountable for, and sometimes supersede the various utilization review mechanisms, such as hospital utilization review committees and state-run peer review programs for Medicaid recipients, that had been built into the three government financing programs. Many PSROs are creatures of county medical societies and preexisting foundations for medical care (FMCs), the latter also set up by county state medical societies.

Controversy has accompanied quality assurance programs, which last year cost in excess of $250 million.[21] The most fundamental criticism is the "fox guarding the henhouse" analogy which questions the wisdom or appropriateness of asking the medical profession to police itself. Putting that argument aside, there is considerable debate over the primary mission of PSROs and what they can reasonably hope to accomplish. One complaint that frequently comes from outside the medical profession is that the PSRO program fails to take into account the patient's perception of what constitutes quality in health care. Within the profession, some say that PSROs' focus on cost has diluted their effectiveness in assessing quality—that they ought to be released from the demands of accounting for costs to focus exclusively on quality of care.[21] Others worry that PSROs may actually elevate costs in some circumstances, by raising a community's standards of care.[22] And still others argue that containing costs is the only capacity PSRO has truly demonstrated, so that this should be viewed as the contribution the program can make. One of the more impartial analyses conducted to date, sponsored by the Institute of Medicine of the National Academy of Sciences, concludes that it is too early to say that hospital concurrent review programs are effective because even where changes in utilization have been documented, the reasons behind them are not fully understood.[20]

Nevertheless, there appears to be a strong movement in industry toward extending the boundaries of quality assurance and utilization review to take in privately financed patients. Business and some labor unions have been arranging for and financing prospective or concurrent peer review of beneficiaries' use of hospitalization, surgery, and many of the newer benefit programs thought especially susceptible to overuse, for example, dental and vision care and hearing aid coverage.

PSROs and FMCs have both formed national umbrella organizations and, according to Kenneth A. Platt of the Colorado Foundation, are ready to implement a national peer review network which hopes to contract with businesses to do utilization review and quality assurance for employees covered under company benefit plans. Continental Airlines has signed up for national peer review of its employees, according to Platt, and "standing in the wings" are similar agreements with several other airlines: United, Western, American, Frontier, as well as other corporations. The review costs the company about $12 to $15 per admission and saves, Platt says, about $1.60 for each $1 spent. The Council on Wage and Price Stability records at least eight major corporations and a large union as having arranged that their beneficiaries' hospital stays be reviewed by medical societies or PSRO-like entities. Responding to more recent inquiries by the Washington Business Group on Health, several corporations reported newly created utilization review programs, including one sponsored by Deere & Company which confronts a delicate problem of implementation sometimes left unaddressed:

There is a provision in Deere's United Auto Workers' contract which allows the company to cease reimbursement within twenty-four hours of a PSRO utilization review determination that medical service is no longer required. Under this provision, however, the patient is "held harmless" and Deere will back him if out-of-pocket payment is demanded by the provider.[23]

Platt makes it quite clear that the PSRO wants no role in mediating such disputes:

> There are still some organizations that are uncomfortable if we rock the boat too hard. So the PSRO has to get an agreement by the company that from the standpoint of medical necessity the PSRO decision is binding. If the company feels the need to take responsibility for social necessity and to continue to fund the case beyond what we have said is medically necessary, that is their prerogative. But we keep a running count of both medically necessary and socially necessary days, because our program's effectiveness is based on the medically necessary days.
>
> Kenneth A. Platt

A member of the conference audience took issue with this approach:

> I understand that if a patient finds himself exceeding your parameters for medically necessary days, he may be the one left holding the bag. It seems to me that the proper way would be to hold the patient blameless and hold the provider responsible for anything like that.
>
> Timothy M. Harrington

Actually there ought not to be an issue of responsibility for disallowed bills, since the concurrent review process should resolve the conflict before the service is rendered. However, the grievance policy in general is an important issue in any program, such as this one, which sometimes puts the patient between two conflicting medical opinions and leaves him to decide what to do.

Apart from issues of implementation, equity, and employee relations, hospital utilization review may be fighting an uphill battle against overwhelming odds in situations with excess hospital beds and powerful incentives on hospital staffs to keep them filled and financed. Still, it was pointed out, peer review is here to stay, is demonstrably effective against at least some costs, and has a contribution to make:

> I am distressed when people speak of peer review at this point as a demonstration project. We're beyond the stage of demonstration— we ought to be talking about rapid escalation. You people in the audience control the bucks and I think you should be aware that there is only a finite period of time in which to bring costs under control or else be faced with externally imposed controls. You are going to have to pay for peer review. It's not free. But for what you get, it is a very very cheap technology.
>
> Eugene McCarthy

On December 15, 1974, the *New York Times* carried an article describing a second surgical opinion program developed in 1972 at the Cornell Medical School in collaboration with several large unions in New York City. Though not the first, the Cornell program has been the best publicized of such programs. Together with published reports of allegedly "unnecessary surgery," including congressional hearings on the subject held in the spring of 1976, the Cornell "success story" has caused second (and third) surgical opinion programs to spread throughout industry at a rate that makes them "probably the fastest growing cost containment measure," in the opinion of the Washington Business Group on Health, and one which may be "gaining acceptance far beyond its proven value."[24]

Second surgical opinion has caught on so rapidly because it appears to be good for both the employer as payer and the employee as patient. Elective surgery represents about 40 percent of hospital admissions for the population under sixty-five, "is the heavyweight component in major medical coverage," for reasons traced by Eugene McCarthy who developed the Cornell program to "a veritable epidemic in elective surgery in the United States". As evidence he cites a 23 percent increase in elective surgery over the past five years, a rate which is four times the growth of the population and which implies that "5 million additional surgical procedures are now being financed by the medical care premium dollar." McCarthy and other health services researchers have come to believe that much of the surgery being done may be unwarranted, a conclusion inferred from significant regional variations in the incidence of certain procedures[25,26] and attributed in part to an oversupply of surgeons,[27] exacerbated by an excess of surgery being done by physicians who are not surgical specialists.[28] The problem of an oversupply of physicians, and especially of surgeons, was a recurrent theme at the Cornell conference (see box pp. 38–39).

Second surgical opinion programs expand the benefit package to enable a patient recommended for elective surgery to seek an independent consultation, usually but not always with a board-certified specialist, as to whether the operation is indicated. If the second opinion conflicts with the first, a third may also be paid for. In some programs the second consultation is voluntary, that is, the patient initiates it; in others the consultation is mandatory, although McCarthy is emphatic that the decision as to which advice to follow must be left to the patient, and that the tie-breaking third opinion ought always to be an option. Second opinion programs normally have an administrative structure (with intake officers who arrange for the second opinion, and a panel of consulting surgeons), and a research orientation which includes provisions to follow the patient's progress for at least a year or two after the episode. Thus they have potential beyond the initial objective of restraining costs and curtailing unwarranted surgery: they increase benefits rather than cutting them back and may improve the information available to the patient-consumer, bringing him back into the decision-making matrix on an important matter related to his health. In addition, they may serve to raise the general standards of care in the medical communities in which they are instituted.

McCarthy's program has run into opposition from the medical profession; others have similarly met resistance.[29] Reporting in the Washington

AN IMPENDING DOCTOR SURPLUS

Ten years ago there was a hue and cry that we needed 50,000 more physicians in the country. The number of medical schools increased from 76 to 115. We are now generating 14,500 physicians a year, compared to ten years earlier when the number was 8,500. By 1984–85, the ratio will be one physician for every 500 people. The implications for industry—buying benefits on behalf of employees in that environment—is staggering. Now we talk about too many hospital beds, but just imagine what we will face as those extra 14,000 physicians per year go into the marketplace in the open-ended entrepreneurial traditional system we have now.

John J. Boardman, Jr., M.D.

We are well oversupplied with surgeons in certain specialities and in certain areas, there's no question about that. Eventually I think, the marketplace will have its impact on surgery; students are already beginning to veer away. But we've got a tremendous problem in the pipeline. The supply machine is still in gear and probably will be for the next decade.

Eugene McCarthy, M.D.

What are all those surgeons going to do, though, all the ones that are being trained?

Richard H. Egdahl, M.D.

Well, if you believe in the marketplace, the word will begin to get around. Why do you think increasing numbers of doctors are going into primary care? Not only the impetus of the federal government but the economic realities. They are seeing the surgeons sitting in there and drinking coffee eight hours a day and operating one and a half. What worries me even more is not just the number of surgeons that we're training, but the number of doctors we're training. What in the devil we're going to do in the mid-1980s with a surplus of doctors, I simply can't imagine.

Kenneth A. Platt, M.D.

If we—that is the appropriate organs of medicine—do not respond, I'll give us only until the early 1980s before the United States will adopt something like the Canadian system where the density of specialists is regulated by area.

Eugene McCarthy, M.D.

One thing we will have to watch are the unanticipated effects of this growing oversupply of doctors. I suspect that this is going to be one of the most powerful inducements to group practice and to closed hospital medical staffs. There may be all sorts of strange side effects of an oversupply of physicians that we don't anticipate. But certainly if the medical marketplace plays itself out in the usual way, we can safely anticipate that one effect we won't see is a reduction of physician fees.

Paul M. Ellwood, Jr., M.D.

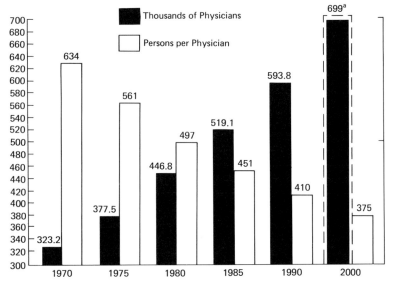

Active U.S. physicians: projected supply and population: physician ratios, 1970–2000. *Sources:* U.S. Department of Health, Education, and Welfare: *Health in the United States 1975 - A Chartbook* (Washington, D.C.: November 1975), p. 20. U.S. Bureau of the Census, Current Population Reports. *Projections of Population of the U.S., 1977–2050.*
a. Projecting a 15% increase for each of the two five-year periods, 1990–2000.

Business Group on Health survey, Corning Glass observed that second opinion programs may be practicable only in large metropolitan areas, and may "lack force in smaller communities. We know from experience that the medical community in our small localities are a close-knit group and tend to take care of each other."[30]

Professional protectionism aside, reservations that objective observers express about second opinion hinge on as yet unanswerable questions about the reasons for the results that have been recorded (for example, what is the range of normal variation in the judgments of qualified physicians under various circumstances?) and the possible long-term effects (will the patients who eluded an operation under the program eventually find their way back into surgery, and if so, with what if any ill effects resulting from this delay?).

McCarthy himself is among the first to admit that the program has uncovered surprises and a few unresolved issues. Over 80 percent of all the participants in his program have accepted the second opinion. Only 17 of 6,500 individuals involved so far have asked for the free tie-breaking third consultation to which the program entitles them. McCarthy finds it surprising that the consultant's opinion carries such weight when the patient has met with him for a total of perhaps twenty minutes. "This is quite a significant factor," he says, "particularly when you think of the so-called physician-patient relationship." In addition, McCarthy points out:

> There is a paradox. Twelve percent of those who were doubly confirmed for surgery have refused the operation. When we looked at this, we found that about 65 percent of those were very, very serious, mostly related to cancer. Surgery is probably medicine's most effective tool in terms of ability to really execute cure in certain diseases, particularly with early diagnosis of cancer. So now we have a challenge, and I think it is one of our major ones, to begin to look at and follow both the confirmed and nonconfirmed cases as to outcome. In fact, the second opinion program may become a technique for recruiting the appropriate individual for surgery.

Whatever the final word on second opinion and other such cost containment programs, McCarthy feels strongly that industry ought to be in the forefront of the effort to implement and analyze them systematically:

> One problem is a common denominator of all of these studies. There is no constituency for cost control in the medical profession at the present time. There are selected leaders and program groups, but by and large no real constituency. The natural constituents for these initiatives are the purchasers of care—trust funds, employers, unions, third-party payers. These are the groups who will have to create the structure within which we can begin to look very critically at cost control.

Judith Lave's endorsement is somewhat more reserved:

PSROs and second surgical opinions don't get at the heart of the problem. PSROs, I believe, have an ambiguous effect. At this point we can only make good guesses as to what their overall effect will be, and my guess is that when their impact becomes clear we will see that they tend to raise costs. Putting surgeons on salary might reduce surgical rates faster than second opinion programs do. This is not to suggest that both programs ought not be implemented— only that they will not have long-term, lasting effect on the overall picture.

Addressing Charges for Services

The third broad group of strategies being employed by industry—those setting out to improve the methods by which providers are reimbursed—is the least widespread and least fully developed of the three classes of activity treated here as part of industry's role as payer. Some businesses and unions are tightening the methods by which they reimburse the hospitals and other facilities, pharmacists, opticians, and optometrists, occasionally even the physicians, serving their beneficiaries. In addition, volume purchasing of pharmaceuticals and blood donor programs have sometimes been implemented successfully and fall within this category.

The relatively primitive state of the art of alternative reimbursement is not for lack of conviction of its importance. To the contrary, rare unanimity emerges among those who have looked at the currently prevailing system of retrospective cost reimbursement of hospitals: it is inflationary. Retrospective reimbursement for actual costs incurred—practiced by Medicare, Medicaid, and many Blue Cross plans—creates a system driven by the antithesis of cost consciousness, where a hospital grows and prospers in direct proportion to the money it can spend. But there, at the problem statement, the agreement abruptly stops, leaving an intractable problem without a good solution. Little is precisely known about the quantitative effects of reimbursement systems or why costs differ widely among hospitals.

Since 1966, when Medicare and Medicaid launched cost-based reimbursement of hospitals on a large scale, incremental steps have occasionally been taken to try to reclaim that skeleton key or, at a minimum, to change some of the locks it fits. The failure of the Medicare "reasonable charge" system is signaled by dramatic geographic differences in the fees that physicians charge. A recent study by the Health Research Group demonstrated that the variations are not explained by differences in cost of living, malpractice premiums, or other professional expenses, quality of care, or supply of or demand for services: "In fact, they appear to result from a payment system which allows physicians in local reimbursement areas to substantially determine their own fees without regard to any of these factors. Thus the system both preserves completely arbitrary regional differences which preexisted Medicare and contains an inherently inflationary bias."[31] Third-party payers have closed doors on certain types of hospital cost (bad debts and research, for example) by excluding them from reimbursement contracts, and the federal government has attempted to place caps or ceilings on reimbursement levels, in the form of wage and price controls, limits on Medicare payments, and, most recently, the Carter administration's proposed cost containment legislation.

On the state and local levels, Blue Cross plans and state governments began in about 1970 to develop hospital rate-setting programs—now numbering roughly twenty-five in twenty-three states and influencing over one-quarter of the nation's hospitals. These have been thoroughly described in a recent review article by Bauer[32] and will not be belabored here.

Large-scale private sector payers for health care have sometimes been able to negotiate prospectively with hospitals or physicians. For example, the United Storeworker's Union Security Plan maintains a panel of physicians who have agreed in advance to accept the plan's schedule of fees. The matter of physicians' fees, and more important, their ordering behavior, is nowhere more frontally addressed than in the prepaid group practice, discussed in detail in chapter 3.

General Motors has been developing prospective reimbursement arrangements with hospitals, and reported to the Council on Wage and Price Stability having reached agreement with twelve hospitals to negotiate annually the rates of payment to apply to corporate employees hospitalized during the year.

> The concept of negotiated budgets has certain inherent problems: I would put negotiated budgets in the category of strategies that have little effect and are likely to have little effect on controlling costs. First, the costs of negotiated budgets are extraordinarily high. Second, the administrator of the hospital whose budget is being established always has the upper hand. He has sufficient information so that he can start high enough to get himself negotiated down to where he wants to be. He's a better player at that game—or she is.
>
> Judith R. Lave

> Isn't the issue, though, really, the fact that in business if our volume is down, we have to cut overhead and that's it. But right away, as soon as hospitals' volume goes down there are proposals to adjust their rates. Isn't the very heart of the problem the fact that hospitals are a protected industry?
>
> Thomas E. Burns

Similar reservations obtain for negotiated physicians' fees unless they are circumscribed within a closed economic system, such as a prepaid health plan. As with many regulatory strategies, clamping down in one area (a single aspect of a physician's practice) simply causes ballooning out in another:

> Any effective cost containment program has got to deal simultaneously with all of the parties and issues involved in the medical care process: consumers, doctors, hospitals, volume, prices, all of them. Attacking one segment at a time inevitably leads to upward adjust-

ments in another segment. And this is true all over the world. In Germany, they regulate physicians' fees, which would be quite a threat to physicians' incomes—except that they have turned to doing more laboratory work in their offices instead. And German physicians are now the highest paid physicians in the world despite a very vigorous effort to control their fees.

Paul M. Ellwood, Jr.

Prospectively determined reimbursement rates raise another issue that is inherent in many cost containment programs—what is to be done about charges that are not covered? The United Storeworkers' Plan handles the problem by circulating to members a list of physicians who have agreed to accept the plan's fee schedule. Members are at liberty to see any physician they wish, but by choosing a physician on the plan's list are assured of receiving full reimbursement.[33] Continental Bank in Chicago has also developed an unusual solution, a "predetermination of benefit" program in which the employee benefit office will advise an employee before he undergoes treatment whether the fee that his physician proposes to charge will be fully covered by his insurance. In essence, the company is providing a translator to decipher both the medical and the insurance industry language for the consumer. "This, then, will eliminate surprise when it is too late to do anything."[34] By implication, the program conveys the message that it is all right to inquire of a physician what his fee will be.

The program initiated by the Storeworkers' Union and the Continental Bank make explicit the communication or consciousness raising function that is to some degree an underlying goal of most of the cost containment efforts sponsored by industry as a payer for care. Better communication—among payers, providers, and consumers—is critically needed in the health system to facilitate informed decisions. On the other hand, it is doubtful that information alone will be sufficient to restore a market in health services. An exceedingly complex set of problems, the defects of the market in health care are attracting increasingly sophisticated attention in both the public and private sectors. In this monograph, the question of competition is treated mostly in conjunction with industry's role as provider of care and sponsor of "alternative delivery systems." Consumer information is touched on in chapter 4 when we look at industry's efforts in the health education sphere. Forthcoming volumes in the Springer Series will explore these questions in depth.

With regard to negotiated fees, it is important to recognize the conflict that arises between the objective of holding down fees on the one hand and of facilitating the flow of information on the other. The Federal Trade Commission (FTC) has recently begun addressing the latter problem by challenging some segments of the medical profession for allegedly fixing prices and restraining trade. The FTC appears not to object to fees set prospectively by groups of payers—only to fees set unilaterally by physician groups. But no one is certain where the lines will be drawn and this confusion may complicate the task of the purchaser of health insurance seeking some measure of control over fees:

For some 20 years, we at General Electric have been trying to use the peer review system in the medical fraternity as a means of setting standards as to the reasonableness of fees. We were very optimistic about these types of standards when we introduced the concept on a major basis in 1955—standards governing both medical care (necessity and quality) and fees (are they usual, customary, and reasonable?) Now, recently, there has been some impairment of that process, I understand, and some question as to the appropriateness of the profession's setting its own fee standards. But if you believe that there ought to be some mechanism by which to judge fees, then who can realistically make those judgments other than peers in the medical community? This is a problem, I think, which is being faced by many plans similar to ours.

C. Stephen Tsorvas

General Electric's problem emanates from conflicting signals on what is to be done to moderate physicians' fees. Conflicts of this nature tend to pervade health policy on two distinct levels. Conflicts over the most effective means to a particular end (for example, equity in physicians' fees) cast doubt on the possibility of finally resolving specific problems in the health care system by engaging in "omnibus tinkering":

We can apply piecemeal controls to the hospitals as we're about to do, to doctors' fees, to length of hospital stay, to elective surgery, to locale of physicians' practices, to CAT scanners, and the like. But my contention is that when we try to get control of one piece at a time, it's likely to be just a bureaucratic nightmare. As a physician, I say we can beat you every time.

Paul M. Ellwood, Jr.

Conflicts over the ends themselves aggravate the situation even further:

Now the problem, the enigma, is how to achieve cost containment in light of competing public policy goals. We want cost control but on the other hand we want greater equity for underserved populations—people in rural and inner city areas, and the poor everywhere. We also want more comprehensive coverage. How can we improve the accessibility and convenience of services to more Americans, while containing costs? That is the fundamental conflict.

Roger M. Battistella

Resolution of the pervasive conflicts is a paralyzing and perhaps unnecessary goal. Instead of arguing over the details of an all-encompassing master plan it may be more important, as Richard Martin suggests, to look carefully at local conditions and do something:

If we in the corporate sector are going to influence health costs and improve the delivery system, we have to get involved and we have to do it properly. The first step is to understand the health delivery system in the communities in which we operate. And then we can use bits and pieces of every strategy we can find (utilization review, altered benefit packages, HMOs and the like)—tailored to the local situation. But without corporate commitment, the job will not be done. And if the private sector fails in this country, there is only one other sector that is going to pick up the ball and that's the federal government.

The temptation for a corporate executive looking at the long list of cost control strategies that are being tried and that may have some merit, is to retreat in dismay. Any one approach alone seems hardly worth pursuing because a substantial commitment of time and energy promises to repay at best a minor impact on the health care cost curve. The time and energy might seem better spent on an activity related directly to the firm's own product or production process. But in Martin's approach there may be an answer. If a number of these strategies are tried thoughtfully and in a cohesive way, it seems reasonable to expect that they could have a very substantial impact not only on the cost curve but on the amount of money the firm actually pays out for health care services.

Industry as Provider: Health Programs Sponsored by Employers or Unions

3

Conditioned to some extent by developments in employee health benefits, but often surprisingly separate, industry's role as a provider of health services has been secondary to the payer role in the resources it has commanded internally and the influence it has wielded externally. But federal legislation and mounting cost pressures in recent years have caused many firms and unions to take a step back and reexamine the provider function. The nature of the changes that seem to be taking place, their origins, the issues they raise, and possible future scenarios will be examined in the volume of background papers and the monograph making up the second and third issues of the Springer Series.

The purpose here is to set the context for those two forthcoming issues by seeking to establish the rough dimensions of industry's role as provider, to sketch the history of some of the central themes, and to relate the provider role to the other activities of industry in the health care system.

Early History

The involvement of industry as a provider of health care for employees goes back at least to the 1870s on the American frontier. Railroading, lumbering, and mining operations in remote areas of the country where medical resources were scarce or nonexistent left employers with little choice in the interest of conserving human capital but to arrange for some fundamental medical services for employees and their families. The quality of the care, however, "did not bear much scrutiny."[1]

Around 1900 a few large companies (Consolidated Edison in New York City, Endicott-Johnson in Johnson City, N.Y., the Homestake Mining Company in South Dakota, and Standard Oil in Louisiana) developed "noteworthy medical programs governing general illness as well as occupational disability. Some of these were administered directly by the employer; some by employer-fostered employee associations. A few covered dependents and occasionally even the community."[1]

Several of the themes that remain central today had already surfaced at this early stage: a tendency on the part of industry to comfortably assume the provider role only when there are obvious gaps in services to be filled; the beginnings of a separate definition for occupational versus nonoccupational medicine; the issue of whether to provide services for employees only, employees and their dependents, or the community at large. These and other key themes resurface repeatedly as the history unfolds.

Meanwhile, the hazards of work in industrial America at the turn of the century were arousing some public attention to the plight of injured workers or the survivors of workers killed in industrial accidents. Recompense was rare and wholly inadequate because the employer was usually able to construct a convincing argument that the mishap had been the consequence of the worker's own carelessness or that of a fellow employee, or that the worker, in taking the job, had willingly assumed whatever risk was involved. Any one of these arguments was normally sufficient defense under the common law.

Reformers in a few states were able to push through legislation improving employees' chances of winning in court, and, indeed, some juries did begin awarding workers more and better settlements. This situation, it is argued,[2] gave rise to the no-fault workmen's compensation system, which has been called a creature of the employers in the same way that the hospital insurance system seems to have emerged to protect the hospitals. Although an insurance system, and thus an element of industry's role as payer for health care, workmen's compensation is a historical antecedent to the field of industrial hygiene—now occupational medicine—and is for that reason discussed here, as background for industry's provider role.

Workmen's Compensation

Economic theory holds that the objective of workmen's compensation laws is to act as a deterrent to accidents or industrially induced disease—that is, an incentive to a safe and healthy work environment—by causing management to internalize the costs of industrial accidents or disease.[3] In fact, it can be-argued, workmen's compensation is a flawed incentive system because it neither returns to the worker the full amount of lost income (usually less than 60 percent) nor ties the insurance premium closely to the injury experience of any but the largest firms.[4] Also, early workmen's compensation laws covered only occupational injuries, and coverage for disease remains inadequate in most cases.

Limitations of the state-administered workmen's compensation system (gaps in workers covered, small cash benefits, delays in administration, high overhead costs, gross discrepancies from one state to another) have been painstakingly dissected in the literature[2,5,6] and at public hearings held by the National Commission on State Workmen's Compensation, created by part of the Occupational Safety and Health Act of 1970. For our purposes here the relevance of workmen's compensation lies in its influence on the development of industry's role as provider of health services. Flawed or not, the system did shift some safety responsibility to the employer and does seem to have stimulated or, at a minimum, accompanied the emergence of industrial hygiene.

Between 1910 and 1920, all but six states had enacted workmen's compensation laws; all fifty now have such a law in force. The usual pattern is for the claims to be insured through private carriers (Ohio, alone of the large industrial states, excludes private carriers from writing workers' compensation insurance), and for the overall program to be administered by state industrial accident boards or commissions. In pursuing the workmen's compensation route, the injured employee usually forgoes all other rights and remedies against the employer. For this reason, workmen's compensation may have legal relevance today to a corporation's malpractice liability as a provider of medical care because it "acts as a buffer to the problem of corporate liability for the negligent conduct of company physicians when a causal connection has been established between work setting and injury."[7] On average, awards tend to cover medical expenses, plus one-half to two-thirds of lost wages.[8] In 1972, thirty-two states had maximum weekly benefits for temporary total disability of less than 60 percent of average weekly wages.[9]

Safety versus Health

The emphasis in workmen's compensation has always been on injury rather than illness. For example, crude estimates (extrapolating New York data nationally) place the number of compensated deaths from occupational diseases in 1971 at under 700, counterposed against the tens of thousands of such fatalities believed to occur each year.[10] The tendency of safety concerns to dominate is a recurrent theme in the history of industrial hygiene. Not until the 1960s, when emerging occupational disease data brought a whole new dimension to the problem of occupational health hazards, did the pendulum begin to swing slowly and partially toward health. As the first official federal recognition of a specific occupational disease, the 1960 Coal Mine Health and Safety Act was an important milestone. The Occupational Safety and Health Act (OSHA) of 1970 (discussed below in some detail) was another, but even OSHA has not eliminated entirely the safety orientation. True, the Occupational Safety and Health Administration has concentrated its standard-setting energies largely on health hazards, but its enforcement activities, through periodic inspections, have been much more vigorously pursued with regard to safety than to health.[11]

Reasons for safety's eclipsing health are easily divined. Accidents are discrete and identifiable events, whereas occupational illness is insidious. The exact etiology of occupational diseases is complex; the diseases have multiple causes and typically take years to develop, have long latency periods, and affect different individuals differently. Information is lacking, for instance, on what constitutes a dangerous chronic exposure to low levels of known toxic substances, not to mention the countless presumably toxic substances whose toxicity has yet to be detected. The National Institute of Occupational Safety and Health (NIOSH) estimates that there are as many as 250,000 chemicals in use today, of which some 12,000 have been identified as toxic. About 2,000 of these are "hazardous materials that may ultimately require development of health standards." So far, as will be discussed below, OSHA has established general exposure limits for 400 but the more complete standards now required by law for only a handful.[12] Little is known about how two or more specific toxic substances might react together in particularly deadly combinations. Health hazards tend to be invisible and thus to require much more difficult and time-consuming inspections than are needed to inspect for violations of safety standards.

Complexities and enigmas notwithstanding, occupational health merits at least as much attention as occupational safety, as evidenced by recent statistics comparing the toll of the two problems: NIOSH estimated in 1975 that at least 4 million workers contract occupational diseases every year, and as many as 100,000 deaths a year may be attributable to occupational disease. On-the-job injuries, by contrast, involve something over 20 million episodes, but account for perhaps 28,000 deaths in a year.[13] Occupational exposure to carcinogens is a vital concern. It is now believed that well over 350,000 Americans die each year of cancer and that "industrial and agricultural technologies are the major contributors in the production of most known environmental carcinogens."[14] Other diseases attributable to work exposures include emphysema, lung fibrosis and other respiratory disorders, deafness, dermatitis, a variety of poisonings, and physiological and psychological stress.

Primary versus Secondary Prevention

Underlying the data on occupational disease is yet another central theme in industrial medicine: the question of where the major payoffs are to be found on the continuum between environmental surveillance, screening, early detection of disease, and medical treatment—in short, where the bulk of available resources ought to be channeled:

> I think employees—and I know unions—are less excited about efforts to prevent a small cancer from becoming a big cancer than

they are about preventing the exposure to the carcinogen. I'd like to see the medical departments of the corporations focused more on real prevention and less on setting up big screening programs that, in effect, use workers as test instruments. We set up a screening program, we point to fifteen people we've found with cancer and then we say we have a preventive program. In the meantime, while we are treating these people and setting up new medical facilities, the hazard still exists and no one does anything about it.

James E. Lapping

Few would disagree that the primary goal ought to be prevention of the initial damaging exposure. The issue arises over *where* and how to intervene in order to prevent occupational disease and to anticipate as yet unidentified problems:

If you think of the various environmentally known diseases that are now obviously present and for which there are government controls, it's not clear how we could have foreseen them before they developed. I don't see how we can effectively take this great multitude of environmental exposures and do any prevention until we actually see clinical cases. And therefore, in the interest of trying to get the biggest bang for the buck we spend, I think that rather than search for the next successor to beryllium disease—whatever that might be—I'd put my preventive bucks up against known problems—common diseases like heart disease and hypertension.

Joseph M. Miller

Questions such as these, involving cost effectiveness and cost-benefit considerations, are a necessary consequence of two relatively new and building pressures: the growing awareness that occupational hazards to health may be extensive and pervasive, tempered by the widespread feeling that the resources available to combat those hazards are finite.[15] The world must have seemed simpler in the early 1900s of the inchoate industrial hygiene movement.

Occupational Medicine Takes Shape

Between 1910 and 1920 the field of industrial medicine emerged in the United States as a firmly established medical specialty. It was part of the occupational safety and health movement that had grown up around the legislative push for workmen's compensation, and also part of industry's preventive apparatus to mitigate potential losses under the new compensation system. Its intellectual roots went back to early eighteenth century Italy and the physician Bernardino Ramazzini, generally recognized as the father of occupational medicine. Ramazzini published a treatise entitled *Diseases of Tradesmen* and counseled his fellow physicians to first ask their patients, "Of what trade are you?"[1] Modern industrial medicine emerged initially from the deplorable working conditions of the industrial revolution in nineteenth century England.

The case is often made that the origins of United States occupational medicine, comingled as they were with workmen's compensation, saddled the profession with a handicap that it has never fully overcome. As the company's representative in workmen's compensation proceedings, in hiring and firing controversies, confidentiality disputes, and other areas of labor-management contention, plant doctors, the argument goes, have been placed in a conflict of interest that greatly complicates the task of establishing a satisfactory physician-patient relationship. This view is forcefully argued by many present-day spokesmen for organized labor, including Glasser of the United Auto Workers[2] and Sheldon W. Samuels of the AFL-CIO: "There is little question in my mind about what most elected union officials [and I suspect most members as well] think of company doctors and the company doctor system. The first and essential view is that company doctors are no less a part of management than the plant engineer, personnel director or the chairman of the board. They are seen as tools of the boss."[3]

Samuels goes on to qualify the statement, suggesting that "some elements of an acceptable patient-physician relationship may often exist. Certainly there is often a reciprocal desire for this to be true." But, he argues, "the plant situation breeds attitudes inimical to the development of a normal patient-physician relationship." Historically, he says, the company, rather than the company doctor is legally responsible for malpractice; "the company doctor has failed to achieve the same degree of self-regulation and institutional protection from exploitation that prevails in the other branches of medicine; most important, he has failed—at least publicly—to establish common cause with the worker on key issues in the plant, in the community or in the legislature."[3]

Moreover, in Samuels's view, confidentiality of patients' records remains a serious problem in industrial medicine, as does the requirement that company medical programs, like other components of corporate structure, justify themselves financially: "Doctors in this position are less likely to be on the worker's side in workmen's compensation cases, definition of environmental conditions affecting health, the impact of the plant on community resources, or the interpretation of preemployment and OSHA-required medical examination. Even when he is, his position in the company usually is not influential enough to balance the arguments of other department heads."[3']

The leadership of occupational medicine is grappling with Samuels' issues. The American Occupational Medical Association last year promulgated a code of ethics (see box pp. 52–53) to guide the profession through the minefield Samuels describes, and has subsequently been debating some of the more intractable problems—having mainly to do with confidentiality and the use of information about workers' health. These questions will be discussed in considerable detail in forthcoming issues of the Springer Series.

On balance, it seems fair to say that although the situation may now be changing, and despite the many dedicated and talented physicians who have made a career of occupational medicine, the field as a whole has been neglected

CODE OF ETHICAL CONDUCT FOR PHYSICIANS PROVIDING OCCUPATIONAL MEDICAL SERVICES

Adopted by the Board of Directors of the American Occupational Medical Association, July 23, 1976

These principles are intended to aid physicians in maintaining ethical conduct in providing occupational medical service. They are standards to guide physicians in their relationships with the individuals they serve, with employers and workers' representatives, with colleagues in the health professions, and with the public.

Physicians should:

1. accord highest priority to the health and safety of the individual in the workplace;
2. practice on a scientific basis with objectivity and integrity;
3. make or endorse only statements which reflect their observations or honest opinion;
4. actively oppose and strive to correct unethical conduct in relation to occupational health service;
5. avoid allowing their medical judgment to be influenced by any conflict of interest;
6. strive conscientiously to become familiar with the medical fitness requirements, the environment and the hazards of the

in medical school curricula and in residency training programs, has been a relatively low prestige choice among the various medical specialties, and has, as a consequence, been isolated in an out-of-the-way niche of medicine, focusing on environmental hazards, and routine treatment of job-related illness and disability.

The intellectual domain of occupational medicine has been likened to a three-legged stool, the legs representing medical science, engineering and chemical sciences, and the social sciences.[4] Within the purview of the industrial physician the primary task has traditionally been monitoring of disease patterns associated with industrial processes and surveillance of the worker's health with an eye to his fitness for the job he is doing and the impact of the job on his health. The specialty focus of occupational medicine emphasizes physical assessment (including general examinations, multiphasic screening, audiometry, cardiovascular stress testing, and similar procedures), toxicology, and epidemiological techniques to gather and analyze data on industrial health work done by those they serve, and with the health and safety aspects of the products and operations involved;

7. treat as confidential whatever is learned about individuals served, releasing information only when required by law or by over-riding public health considerations, or to other physicians at the request of the individual according to traditional medical ethical practice; and should recognize that employers are entitled to counsel about the medical fitness of individuals in relation to work, but are not entitled to diagnoses or details of a specific nature;

8. strive continually to improve medical knowledge, and should communicate information about health hazards in timely and effective fashion to individuals or groups potentially affected, and make appropriate reports to the scientific community;

9. communicate understandably to those they serve any significant observations about their health, recommending further study, counsel or treatment when indicated;

10. seek consultation concerning the individual or the workplace whenever indicated;

11. cooperate with governmental health personnel and agencies, and foster and maintain sound ethical relationships with other members of the health professions; and

12. avoid solicitation of the use of their services by making claims, offering testimonials, or implying results which may not be achieved, but they may appropriately advise colleagues and others of services available.

problems. Very little material on industrial medicine is taught in standard medical school curricula; specialists generally receive postgraduate training in schools of public health.

Until very recently, the proper scope of occupational medicine has been closely circumscribed to exclude involvement in care of illness or injury with nonoccupational origins. The distinction between medical problems that are job-related and those that are independent of work is often difficult to draw, but the organized medical profession has long insisted on the distinction. The Conference Board found, in a survey of industrial health programs, that "company programs, and company policy statements are often largely a rephrasing of" American Medical Association positions, which have been "major influences on the scope and character of company programs."[5] The AMA's amended policy statement, adopted in 1971, asserted that with certain limited exceptions, "treatment of nonoccupational illness and injury has been and is not now ordinarily considered to be a routine responsibility of an occupational health program."[6] This amendment represented a significant loosening of earlier strictures against nonoccupational involvement, but physicians and executives in industry are for the most part, still chary of invading the medical profession's private "turf."

Moreover, there is debate over the possible impact on occupational medicine of moving it into the general medical care system. Some argue that such a move would completely overshadow any occupational health concern whatever,[7] and worry that the need for resources for acute care would predominate over the less immediate need for preventive occupational programs, as allegedly did occur in Britain with implementation of the National Health Service.[8] Others believe that the only way to upgrade occupational medicine is to bring it into the mainstream of good primary care.[9] In either case, there appears to be an acute shortage of occupational physicians, along with under-supplies of most other types of occupational health professionals.[10,11] NIOSH estimates that 28,000 full- and part-time physicians are needed by industry to comply with OSHA and that about 13,000 are currently practicing full- or part-time.[12] General physicians in the community, moreover, are believed to be seriously uninformed on the rudiments of occupational medicine:[13]

> The problem I see for our company, which has numerous large and small plants, is that especially where we have small plants we cannot economically justify a full-time physician on the staff. But even in Columbus, Indiana, a town of 52,000 which has a fine concentration of specialists in the various medical fields, these physicians are not well enough acquainted with the problems of occupational medicine. So when we refer employees out even for minor occupational complaints, we literally have had to play the role of the instructor and by careful and diplomatic persuasion to maintain good relationship to get the outside physicians to do what we want them to do, and yet maintain the dichotomy between occupational care and private medicine.
>
> Harold Richmond

On the credit side of the ledger, it can be argued that occupational medicine is now in some respects a discipline whose time has come. The public health and preventive medicine orientation that it has traditionally had are attaining new prominence in medical circles with an emerging concensus that medical care per se may be less likely in the future to influence broad patterns of morbidity and mortality than will general efforts to promote health and prevent illness (see chapter 4). Though sometimes felt by labor to be excessive, the emphasis in industrial health programs on considerations of cost may be convertible into an asset as cost control in health care becomes a widely accepted societal goal.

From a public health perspective, occupational medicine has several intrinsic advantages and presents some unique challenges. First, over 80 million American men and women spend over one-quarter of their lives in a workplace outside of the home. The health of these people is affected by their work, probably to a much greater extent than is now known, and at their places of work they are especially accessible to public health interventions. Occupational medicine can theoretically serve as an entry into the medical system for people who have been on the outside. In that regard, occupational medicine is analogous to school health or family planning services, and, like those programs, addresses a segment of society whose health "is vitally important and is peculiarly at risk."[14] Of course to function effectively as an entry to the external health care system, the occupational medical department needs some formal linking mechanism so that patients are not only referred to the outside but are also followed effectively.

In a public health sense, the substantial opportunity for prevention of disease, disability, and death among the age group and social class represented by the wage earner is also important. Occupational medicine has always offered the opportunity for preventive approaches to large populations; industry has substantial accumulated experience in running certain types of preventive programs (alcoholism and drug abuse programs, in some cases, health education, and periodic screening programs). There is now evidence that this experience is being recognized and built upon by the profession, and that the worksite is being viewed as a natural locus for a range of preventive medicine approaches.

The Occupational Safety and Health Act

Much of the impetus for occupational medicine's reassessment and expansion and for industry's changing perception of its role in health care is coming from the Occupational Safety and Health Act of 1970 (P.L. 91-596). Heralded by Senator Yarborough, its Senate sponsor, as "one of the truly great landmark pieces of social legislation in the history of the country,"[1] OSHA passed both houses of Congress with only eight dissenting votes and became law on April 28, 1971. The legislative history of the act is well documented by Ashford[2] and, from a different perspective, by a Nader study group.[3] Smith recently published a careful evaluation study of the act's impact to date[4] and the federal government publishes annual presidential reports on occupational safety and health, along with a steady stream of educational and informational material.

The stated purpose of OSHA is "to assure safe and healthful working conditions for working men and women." The act created several new governmental bodies with responsibilities exclusively for occupational safety and health: within the Department of Labor, an Occupational Safety and Health Administration (OSHA), charged with establishing and enforcing standards; within the Department of Health, Education, and Welfare, a National Institute on Occupational Safety and Health, to serve as the scientific arm of the operation and to assist in developing the criteria documents on which OSHA could base its standards. In addition, the act created a three-member Occupational Safety and Health Review Commission as an independent adjudicatory agency to which aggrieved employers can bring their complaints about OSHA enforcement actions, and a National Advisory Committee on Occupational Safety and Health with membership representing the public, management, labor, and safety and health professionals, whose job is to advise the secretaries of labor and of health, education, and welfare on the implementation of the act. Advisory committees on specific topics of concern were also provided for in the act; standing committees on construction safety and health and agriculture have been created, as well as ad hoc committees on marine terminal facilities, hazardous materials labeling, and coke oven emissions.

The act applies to any United States employer who is engaged in business affecting interstate commerce—over 4.1 million employers of some 57 million workers. It establishes a "general duty" on the part of every employer to furnish a work environment that is "free from recognized hazards that are causing or likely to cause death or serious physical harm," and requires every employer to comply with the standards promulgated by OSHA.

The process of setting standards envisaged by the act is graduated, with interim standards to be published within the first two years of implementation and fuller standards to be promulgated through a complex administrative procedure (involving twenty-two steps within the bureaucracy as well as public hearings and initial research)[5] as the secretary of labor becomes convinced of their necessity. In the first two years, OSHA set 4,400 interim standards, nearly half of which came from preexisting voluntary standards of the American National Standards Institute (ANSI) and the National Fire Protection Association (NFPA). The remainder derived from federal standards previously established through the Walsh-Healey Act, the Construction Safety Act, and the Longshoremen's and Harbor Workers Compensation Act. Of the interim standards, 2,100 apply to all industry and the rest only to the construction and maritime trades. OSHA's interim standards occupy 800 pages in the *Code of Federal Regulations*.

For many of the abovementioned reasons that workers' compensation has emphasized safety over health, the interim OSHA standards had a decided safety cast. Preestablished standards on which there was adequate consensus were much more common in the less ambiguous safety sphere than in industrial health. In recent years, however, OSHA has striven to focus on the setting of health standards, and has found the political atmosphere charged.

The process of setting health standards has engendered much legal and political acrimony. OSHA has set standards for fourteen carcinogenic chemicals used in various industries including the chemical and plastics industries, in the manufacture of dyes and pigments, and in the preparation of flame-resistant fabrics. These were published in the *Federal Register* in January 1974 and have been the subject, before and since their publication, of bitter contention and several court cases with the Oil Chemical, and Atomic Workers International Union and the Health Research Group calling them inadequate and the chemical manufacturers' industry calling them overly stringent. In setting standards for asbestos and vinyl chloride and for pesticides, OSHA has experienced similar difficulties. As a consequence, OSHA's activities have been much in the news, seldom with a favorable coloration.

The controversy roiling around OSHA may be inevitable, given the charged atmosphere into which it emerged. This possibility is suggested by Ashford's recent book analyzing that atmosphere:

> Health, work, and environment rank among the most important areas of social concern today, and the point where these concerns converge—the workplace—has become a microcosm of national conflict. Not only are issues directly related to the long-neglected field of occupational health and safety receiving increased attention, but the nation is beginning to perceive that some of its larger concerns may be centrally connected to the workplace. For example, the growing debate over health care and preventive medicine cannot proceed far without encountering the probable occupational causation of a surprising proportion of disease. Problems of industrial productivity, work alienation, and management-labor disputes relate increasingly to occupational health and safety. In addition, the monetary costs of job injury and disease are beginning to be more fully realized and deserve closer attention during a period of inflation and of materials and energy shortages.[6]

Ashford goes on to enumerate "four kinds of conflict characterizing health and safety in the work environment": (1) the clashing of different self-interests that is typical of labor-management relations in many issues; (2) conflicts derived "from an insufficient data base;" (3) conflicts arising out of "differences in perceptions as to what is fair and just in public policy;" and finally, (4) conflicts relating to the fact that various institutions and forces in society, which ought to have common interests and concerns in workers' health and safety, are often poorly coordinated or even functioning at cross purposes. Smith encapsulates the fundamental disagreement as a question of "how much safety and health" the government can properly mandate, and at what point should economic feasibility come into play as a qualifier to the mandate for absolute safety.[4]

If OSHA's difficulties are far-reaching, so too is its potential impact on occupational safety and health generally and specifically on industry-sponsored health services, which is the focus here. The specific impact emanates largely from the health standards, which tend to prescribe not only the work practices and controls (contamination control procedures, personal protective equipment, industrial hygiene) needed to protect employees from the hazards, but also the medical surveillance, employee education, and data collection and reporting that have been the traditional functions of industrial medical departments. As the permanent standards are promulgated, they will certainly continue to increase the responsibilities of affected industries (those using the cited substances in their production processes) to monitor the health of their employees. Conceivably, this could lead over time to a spillover effect to employees not directly exposed to hazards·

> *OSHA has had an enormous impact in broadening management interest in medical care beyond the limits of OSHA. I see many corporations today who say: Because of the OSHA standard, we*

have to examine these people who are exposed to this particular hazard. But in equity, we must then go and examine people who are not exposed to that hazard because we don't want to set up a two-tiered system.

Stanley P. de Lisser

OSHA has already had a discernable impact in more sophisticated health and safety demands at the collective bargaining table; recent contract negotiations have included specific provisions aimed at improving job safety and health. In addition, the stepped-up medical surveillance of workers mandated by OSHA standards has led and will surely continue to lead to the discovery of hitherto unsuspected occupational and nonoccupational health problems:

I think one of the greatest implications of OSHA will be the uncovering of nonrelated medical problems in the course of an OSHA-required examination. I have been involved with the implementation of the Mining Safety Act of 1969, which certainly has brought to light many other health problems unrelated to black lung disease among those coal miners living in underserved areas of Appalachia. More recently I've been involved with health screening examinations pursuant to coke emission standards which went into effect on January 20, 1977. Again we are uncovering a whole Pandora's box of serious medical problems. And the real question is, what do we in industry plan to do about these findings?

Joseph M. Miller

I think we have an obligation to capitalize on the momentum achieved by OSHA —to use government regulations and labor demands as our two most prominent allies as we seek to push management in companies that have not done an adequate job of safeguarding employees health and providing for health care management. The challenge will be to develop convincing arguments (and I don't know what they are) to show management that upgrading their health services for employees will enable them to save costs over the long run.

Stanley P. de Lisser

These cost-benefit issues will be difficult to think through, especially with regard to occupational disease with its deferred onset. It may not be possible to prove that the individual firm's interest as contrasted to a general societal interest is best served by the required investment to mitigate occupational disease.

Of particular import for employer-sponsored health services will be the leveling effect OSHA could have, forcing the smaller industries or those that are large but geographically dispersed to catch up to some extent with the large industries that have for thirty to forty years been supporting medical departments which provide sophisticated occupational medical and safety services to employees. "These departments cover only about 25 percent of the nation's workers," according to a statement by the AMA's Council on Occupational Health, which asserted that "the challenge of the present situation is to extend these benefits to small business and industry and to the workers in millions of enterprises who lack such programs."[7]

Tom Herriman of the Amalgamated Clothing and Textile Workers Union asserts that the size of the firm or industry is not the only decisive factor:

> There are large industries that don't provide much medical care to their employees. The textile industry is an example: it employs around a million people in the United States and has some serious occupational safety and health problems. Many of the largest companies in that industry do nothing at all in the way of routine medical care; most do little or no screening to see if people are developing occupational diseases. It's not just a question of size or concentration because I'm speaking now of plants where there may be 1,000 to 2,000 workers, which ought, I think, to be enough to justify some kind of program. The apparel industry is a little different because it involves much smaller factories and shops, creating a different set of problems. I certainly hope that OSHA will cause screening programs to become much more prevalent than they are now in the textile and apparel industries.

Another kind of leveling function that OSHA can perform harks back to the economic theory underlying workmen's compensation laws. While the objective of workmen's compensation was to internalize the cost of accidents or illnesses caused by the job environment, OSHA seeks to anticipate the problems by requiring internalization of the costs of prevention. Since diminishing environmental hazards can be a very costly proposition, the firm's competitive position in the marketplace could suffer as a consequence, unless everyone in the competitive mix is required to assume similar responsibilities. In effect, that is the statement OSHA seeks to make. Ashford points out that requirements to diminish occupational hazards are more onerous on small firms and firms with smaller profit margins than for larger or more profitable ones. The cheapest control technologies are available only on a large scale and technical assistance on how best to institute controls is expensive. He predicts that consistent enforcement over the long run could cause "an encouragement of new technology, substitute materials, and redesigned jobs that should result in higher productivity, decreased worker absenteeism, and improved job health and safety."[8]

The final and perhaps most important long-range influence on industry-sponsored health services of OSHA—and of the changing perceptions of occupational disease that shaped OSHA—has been a blurring of the lines traditionally separating occupational and nonoccupational health care. Those lines had been firmly drawn by the American Medical Association, had been adhered to by occupational physicians and deferred to by industrial executives. Reporting on a 1971 survey, the Conference Board noted skepticism on the part of corporate executives about increased company involvement in nonoccupational health care, and cited six reasons. The first was "deference to what many management executives, and many occupational physicians as well, regard as the economic or marketing rights of private physicians."[9]

The quotations presented in the box attest to the fact that these feelings do still exist among occupational physicians but are beginning to fade. The change reflects pressures from OSHA and the rising cost of the benefit package—"the greatly changed stake of employers in the health of their employees as a result of benefit programs,"—which "has stimulated management interest in the question whether, and in what degree, it may be to its advantage to fill some of the gaps and weaknesses in community health care by initiating, or broadening, in-house programs of primary care."[10]

It is here that the payer and provider roles begin again to converge, having diverged around 1911 when health and disability insurance began to replace in-plant medical services as a lower-cost alternative.[11] Now unable to control rising costs on the benefits side of the equation, industry is beginning to wonder if more active involvement in the services side might not have an effect. But the correspondence between the two is complex and the potential for impact elusive. For example, a company that is paying, in a year, $760 per employee for health benefits and $20 per employee for in-house health services, cannot realistically hope to shift $5 per employee directly from the

---

Occupational Medicine Redraws Its Boundaries

Gilbeart H. Collings: It is important to understand the history behind occupational medicine. Until very recently the fundamental concept that there is a vast and absolute distinction between things which are related to job and things which are not related to job had pervaded our thought and action. With almost religious fervor, occupational medicine tried to stay out of those things which were not related to jobs. The distinction between occupational and nonoccupational was the daily grist of occupational medicine, often winding up in litigation to determine whether a condition was caused by job or was not and therefore, in the mind of the occupational physician, whether it was in his legitimate province or that of those other guys out there in the community. Also, the medical profession generally has regarded occupational medicine as a kind of a bastard stepchild off there in never never land. It's going to take us a long time to get over that because it is deeply ingrained. Although it's perfectly obvious if you look at it from a logical standpoint that the definitional boundaries between occupational and nonoccupational are not only disappearing, they

benefit to the service side. The payoff, if any, would probably be deferred and would be difficult if not impossible to isolate from the welter of intervening variables influencing employees' health status and the cost of employee health care.

The subtleties and complexities of the equation are not lost on management; still, there does seem to be, in the larger corporations and industries, an openness to experimentation and to the possibility of assuming some kind of self-administration of health services analogous to self-administration of health insurance. A few of the potential models are already being developed and tested by expanding existing corporate in-house programs, linked variously to the external health care system, and occasionally (as in corporately developed prepaid plans) bringing the benefit package into a closed system of services and financing.

Industrial Medical Programs

Most large corporations and some smaller ones have long sponsored at least a rudimentary in-house clinic to handle minor illness and injury on the job. The occupational medical program is considered to have a dual mission:

probably were never there in the first place because there's not very much you can point out to me that is solely occupational, or solely nonoccupational.

Joseph M. Miller: I think one serious obstacle to innovation still remains, namely the medical profession itself as represented by practicing physicians. Because the private practitioner of medicine out there, I think, still sees occupational medicine as a potential adversary to his economic livelihood.

Leon J. Warshaw: I am convinced that the conflict with the practicing profession is much less of a problem today. When the AMA set that sharp dividing line between occupational and nonoccupational, they viewed industrial medicine as a potential intrusion on the economic prerogatives of the private practitioner. I believe that's no longer the case. We must cross the bridge between occupational health and the external health care system. We've moved beyond the early famous stories about the occupational physician who wouldn't treat the guy who had a heart attack in the plant. That's gone. We must now begin to start to get into real congruence between the occupational health system and the external medical care system.

environmental surveillance of the workplace for potential agents of disease or injury, and medical surveillance of the work force for susceptibility thereto. Sometimes the environmental "industrial hygiene" functions are separate from the programs administered by the medical director; sometimes they are under his purview. Typically, services are provided through on-site primary care clinics staffed by full-time or part-time physicians and/or occupational nurses, or through contractual or referral ties with the external fee-for-service medical care system.

The scope of services ranges widely but traditionally involves some combination of preemployment medical examinations, health surveillance and screening, health education, diagnosis and treatment of occupational or nonoccupational illness or injury, counseling, and referral for outside care. Specialized programs are common: hypertension, alcoholism, and drug-abuse control, weight reduction and smoking clinics, immunization campaigns, or first aid and safety education. Under OSHA's influence multiphasic health testing methods are said by the Washington Business Group on Health to be spreading rapidly through industry.[1] These vary widely, but usually involve some automation of the test procedures and the processing of results.[2,3] There has been an ongoing debate in the medical literature over the value of health screening programs. There seems to be concensus that any screening that is done ought to be specifically targeted by age, sex, and risk factors. Breslow and Somers' recent proposal in the *New England Journal of Medicine* for a lifetime health monitoring program illustrates such an approach.[4]

Industry-sponsored health services have been offered as a convenience to employees and in the hope of reducing time away from work. Executive health programs are frequently more extensive than those for rank-and-file employees. Assumptions about the relative cost effectivness of different programs are common, but true cost-benefit analysis is rare,[5,6] as is systematic measurement of outcomes.

Labor unions, too, have long been providers of health services,[7] sometimes in multiunion groups, sometimes in conjunction with management, as for example, through a Taft Hartley trust. The first union health center was established in 1913 by the International Ladies Garment Workers' Union in New York City; as of the last count known to us (1969) there were 101 union health centers serving 1.6 million members.[8] The range and scope of services provided and the extent of eligibility vary widely from one union clinic to the next. Union-run clinics have encountered numerous problems, often including low utilization[9] and serious resource constraints.[10] They seem unlikely to expand conspicuously in the near future. As a matter of policy, organized labor is looking to national health insurance for long-range solutions to workers' problems of access to health services, with supplementary activities in some areas in organizing and working with prepaid group practices, as elaborated below.

Corporate-sponsored health programs were thoroughly examined in a 1974 Conference Board report summarizing the results of a 1971 survey of the status and scope at that time of health services provided by over 800 large

corporations (all having at least 500 employees).[11] The report compared its
1971 findings with results obtained a decade earlier and found, overall, that
changes in expenditures for or staffing of employee health care were relatively
minor. A sizable minority of firms reported introducing new services—pre-em-
ployment screening had spread from 63 percent to 71 percent of employers
surveyed; work-related periodic exams from 40 percent to 53 percent; general
periodic exams from 39 to 57 percent. Among the 30 percent employing a full-
or part-time physician, 85 percent reported that they did provide some diagnostic or treatment services for conditions not resulting from the job. There are
no available data with which to update this profile of employer-sponsored
health care but impressionistic evidence, such as that collected by the Council
on Wage and Price Stability and the Washington Business Group on Health,
strongly suggests a marked change in the trend since 1971. Nevertheless, many
of the results of the Conference Board survey and the accompanying narrative
are still entirely relevant. For example, the variables that were found to corre-
late with a firm's expenditures for employee health care have probably not
changed appreciably. The survey found a "disproportionately high percentage
of manufacturing firms and a disproportionately low percentage of wholesaling
and retailing firms" to be "high spenders." The largest companies tended to be
higher spenders, as did the firms with higher per employee earnings: two-
thirds of companies with 50,000 or more employees and half of those earning
$4,000 per employee before taxes were in the higher spending category.[11]
OSHA has introduced some new variables—the nature of the production
process and the substances used therein—that will certainly influence employers' investments in health care and will be interesting to monitor.

The Conference Board report, together with the next two issues of the
Springer Series, will provide the interested reader with substantial detail on
the nature of health services provided in industrial medical clinics, the issues
they face, and the prospects for expansion. The present discussion is, therefore,
limited to industry's involvement in developing "alternative delivery systems," particularly prepaid health plans or HMOs.

Creating Alternative Delivery Systems—A Role for Industry

As the benchmark for a discussion of alternative delivery systems, it may
be useful to ask, alternative to what—what is the present system and which of
its features are considered most in need of changing? Largely, it is solo
practice, with physicians earning fees for individual services and with third-
party financing paying the lion's share of the bill. It is technologically oriented
and probably oversupplied with hospital beds, at least in some areas. It is
complicated by a medical malpractice crisis—in terms of premiums—that is
said to grossly drive up the ordering of tests and other high-cost items justified
by "defensive medicine." And the reimbursement system seems to be seriously
flawed, leading to a relative lack of structure in the delivery system.

Under the traditional plan, you, that is, usually, the employer, negotiate into a set of benefits or dollars, whichever you do, and then you go to the carrier and try to get your best deal in terms of what the dollars will buy or how the benefits are administered. In any case, what you say to your employees, in effect, is we have this set of benefits, this is your carrier, here is your ticket, now you find your way through this system. You find your primary care physician—your internist—and you get your own referrals to specialists as you need them.

John J. Boardman, Jr.

The best known alternative delivery system is the one Boardman represents, the prepaid health plan, or health maintenance organization (HMO):

The essential difference that distinguishes a prepaid group practice program from the traditional arrangement is that the prepaid plan undertakes to provide or arrange for the provision of hospital and professional services and guarantees their availability 365 days a year, twenty-four hours a day.

Officially, a health maintenance organization is "an organized health care delivery system which provides a wide range of comprehensive health care services to a voluntarily enrolled population in exchange for a fixed and prepaid periodic payment.[12] Coined in a 1971 article by Paul Ellwood and associates,[13] the "HMO" label acquired a Federal imprimatur in the 1973 Health Maintenance Organization Act (P.L. 93-222). A more accurate descriptor is "prepaid health plan" because the programs' essence has more to do with the fiscal and management controls dictated by a fixed annual budget than with maintaining health.

Within the confines of the general definition above, prepaid health plans come in two basic forms, each susceptible of various permutations. Best known is the closed-panel prepaid group practice (PPGP), in which member physicians earn a salary or a capitation-based fee with or without a bonus, and practice in a multispecialty ambulatory care center, usually equipped with supportive services such as laboratories and x-ray facilities, sometimes including medical auxiliaries and other nonphysician health professionals. Except in emergency situations, enrollees are covered only for services obtained through the prepaid system and have to pay out of pocket for "out-of-plan" care.

The second major prototype is the foundation-model or independent practice association (IPA)-HMO. Here the participating physicians continue to practice in their individual offices and to receive fees for services rendered. These are drawn from a fund made up of capitation payments from a centrally administered fund which in turn is financed through premiums paid by enrollees. The prepaid group practice plan is "capitation in (from subscribers) and salary out (to providers)," the IPA, "capitation in and fee for service out." IPAs evolved from county and state medical society–sponsored foundations for medical care.[14] Typically, IPAs practice peer review according to preestablished standards of practice, and place member physicians "at risk" at least for their own services, and occasionally for hospitalization and drugs, should the capitation funds be exhausted before the end of the year. The physician members of an IPA-HMO continue to maintain a substantial practice that is outside of the plan. Physician risk-sharing for all services makes sense because orders that physicians write—notably for prescription drugs and hospitalization—directly account for more than half the nation's total expenditures for health care. Sharing the risks for inefficient operations presumably encourages more frugal ordering habits.

Some prepaid group practice plans have unequivocally demonstrated the ability to reduce members' hospitalization rates and thereby to save some costs, without evidence of compromised quality. Since hospitalization consumes about 40 cents of the nation's health care dollar, it is widely acknowledged as a prime target for cost control. In fact, the prepaid group practice experience with hospitalization is often cited as evidence that the general population could get by spending many fewer days in hospital beds than is now common practice. As one gets into making comparisons of hospitalization experiences under different plans, it is important to look for differences in the populations being served. Age, for example, ought to be corrected for because the elderly appropriately use more medical services than does the general population. The potential of IPAs to reduce hospitalization is not clear:[15,16]

> There's no question that our IPA programs are producing the same types of results as the closed-panel approach. As a matter of fact, we're better than many of the closed-panel programs. We're approaching Kaiser in days of hospitalization per 1,000 enrollees, and we're satisfied with that. From about 800 to 469 days per 1,000 over a five-year period of time isn't too bad. The key to its success lies with the complete acceptance and cooperation of the physicians. There's no question about control. You can go to any one of our programs and talk to the physicians—it's their plan.
>
> Jacob J. Spies

> It depends on the IPA, I suppose. One of the seven HMOs in the Minneapolis–St. Paul area is the Hennapin County Medical Society's IPA, composed of 1,100 physicians. I'm a little concerned about what type of controls exist when you have that many physicians utilizing seventeen or eighteen hospitals.
>
> John J. Boardman, Jr.

IPAs do avoid some of the initial problems that closed-panel plans have encountered. Start-up costs for closed-panel HMOs are high. Building the ambulatory care center can drive the initial costs to $3 million to $5 million for a new program serving 30,000 to 50,000 people.[17] The self-sustaining level of membership at which the program can begin to meet operating costs out of the prepaid insurance premium is estimated at about 30,000 to 40,000 members,[17] so early enrollment experience can be critical, and has often been a problem.

There are certain costs in pulling a medical group together and building a facility. The important thing, though, is being able to correctly assess the market—what size it will be and how quickly it will be penetrated. The development costs have been a problem for prepaid group practices, largely, I believe, because their organizers have not adequately understood their markets.

John J. Boardman, Jr.

Though perhaps less efficient, the IPA variation requires a smaller start-up investment and tends to be more attractive to physicians. Most of the existing IPAs were created by organized medicine in response to the threat of closed-panel plans' being started in the community. Enlisting enrollees in an IPA is facilitated by the large panel of participating physicians, increasing the likelihood that the new subscriber can continue under the plan with his previous personal physician:

In all our plans, we require that 75 percent of the eligible individuals accept the HMO option or we won't write the HMO in that particular area. We have never failed to get 75 percent because in developing a program, an IPA first makes certain that as many as possible of the community physicians are involved. As you get into marketing the IPA, you can present a list of participating physicians, preferably including the individual's own family doctor, thereby preserving the patient-physician relationship. In many instances patients who fail to find their own physicians on the list will ask them why they're not participating in the program. In Milwaukee, for example, the fact that 1,000 out of approximately 1,250 actively practicing physicians in that city are participants in the IPA can be attributed to pressure not only from their colleagues but from their patients as well.

Jacob J. Spies

Prepaid plans differ also in their relationships with the hospital or hospitals to which their members are sent: Kaiser-Permanente Health Plan, the largest HMO, owns most of the hospitals to which its members go; most prepaid plans are "at risk" for hospitalization, that is, they arrange for and finance it through the capitation fees; a few, such as the Health Insurance Plan of New York, cover ambulatory care but require other coverage, through a supplementary plan, for inpatient hospital care. Diversity is found also in the financial structure of prepaid plans—whether they are voluntary, nonprofit, proprietary, or cooperative—and, finally, in the aegis under which they operate—physician groups, hospitals, consumer groups, public agencies, medical schools, insurance carriers, organized labor, or business.

Industry has had a continuous but variable involvement in the half-century history of prepaid health plans. The early contract medicine of the frontier enterprises (railroading, mining, and the like) was a form of prepaid plan, and its questionable quality can be blamed for a stigma that "packaged medicine" has had difficulty escaping. Private industry was behind the creation of by far the largest and best known HMO in the nation, the Kaiser-Permanente Health Plan, originally established in California and now also operating in Oregon, Cleveland, Denver, and Hawaii:

> *Our organizational history goes back to the depths of the Depression. Effectively we are the child of a large industrial empire—Kaiser Industries. Originally, the program started because there was a need to provide medical services first in remote construction sites and then, during the war, in an urban area. At the outset the program served only employees of the various Kaiser companies. In 1946, with the cessation of hostilities, Kaiser Industries shrunk dramatically and many former employees in the Bay Area asked if they could continue in the program. Starting with approximately 10,000 members in 1946, today the Kaiser Foundation Health Plan serves some 3 million.*
>
> John J. Boardman, Jr.

The Kaiser story has been recounted many times[18] and is important here chiefly to illustrate the role industry can play in developing prepaid plans. Although completely separate from the company, the Kaiser Foundation Health Plan grew out of employees' needs for care in medically underserved areas and the intense personal interest of Henry J. Kaiser, carried on by his son Edgar. Since those pioneering days, there have been creative examples of industry leadership in community efforts to establish prepaid health plans—Minneapolis–St. Paul is a frequently cited case[19]—but little until very recently to suggest that the few examples were more than interesting but anomalous wrinkles in the history of industry roles in health care. In part, this desultory growth reflects setbacks in the HMO movement generally. Professor T. E. Chester from Manchester, England, queried the speakers at the Cornell conference about the reasons for slow growth of HMOs:

> *I have listened with great interest to the high praise you have for HMOs. But I can't help remembering that this concept has been around for quite some time and yet HMOs still cover only a very small proportion of your population. What puzzles me is that if it is such an excellent system, why has it not become a true alternative? What have been the impediments to growth? Because, proceeding at the present rate, it will be the year 3000 before it will cover your country.*

HMO advocates blame political vicissitudes for stalling the growth of their movement. In a February 1971 "health strategy message" President Nixon endorsed the concept of the HMO as a promising vehicle for containing rising health care costs. But by the time that sentiment had been converted to legislation in the 1973 HMO Act, a peculiar alliance of conservative forces in organized medicine and liberal forces seeking to make HMOs a panacea had forged a piece of stultifying "enabling legislation."[20]

The act set qualification standards that were unreasonably stringent. For example, to qualify in the program an HMO had to offer a comprehensive package of services, including such things as opthalmology, mental health, and dentistry for children. Open enrollment periods were required for thirty days out of each year, when members of the community had to be admitted to the plan on a first come, first served basis, regardless of health status. Community rating of subscription fees was required. The attractive features for qualifying under the act included some federal start-up support and the right, under a "dual choice" provision, to demand marketing access to companies in the service area with twenty-five or more employees. In October 1976 Congress amended the 1973 HMO Act to provide greater flexibility to HMOs in their design and operation.[21] In the meantime, however, progress had been impeded. Observes Boardman:

> One of the greatest inhibitors to HMO development was the passage of the HMO Act. Some of us who have been in this business for quite a while like to say that the HMO used to be a lot of fun until the government decided to get involved. Since that time it's been much more difficult.

At the same time the HMO Act was muddying the waters, Boardman contends, the major insurance carriers in the country—those with the where-withal to stimulate innovation in alternative delivery systems—were diverted from this activity by the spate of national health insurance proposals, starting in the early 1970s, which turned insurers' attention to the problem of how to preserve a role in a nationally financed health system. And finally, he believes, business might have been more inclined to experiment with alternatives as a means of containing the costs of the health benefit package had it not been for the false signals produced by the economic stabilization program:

> With the imposition of controls in the summer of 1971, the medical care component of the consumer price index began to drop down and parallel the remainder of the index. People were fooled during that nearly three-year period of controls and it was not until the controls were lifted in April 1974 that hospital and physician charges began to rise again and industry began to recognize what had been, all along, a sleeping giant.

It remains to be seen whether industry will now move aggressively into promoting and sponsoring HMOs. Boardman's organization, Kaiser-Perma-nente Advisory Services hopes so:

> There should be a corporate posture toward the development of a delivery system. Over the last eighteen to twenty-four months, corporations have begun to wrestle with the notion that health care costs should no longer be regarded as inevitable, like death and taxes; that instead there are ways they can intervene in the system. They begin with such things as innundating hospital boards, Health Systems Agencies, Blue Cross–Blue Shield, and after your

frustrations have been heightened at that level, moving to intro-
duce alternative delivery systems. The administrative controls, the
benefits manipulation are all important. But the critical element,
as I see it, is that the corporate community, both from a financial
and a management standpoint, has to be the catalyst in trying to
get some sort of alternative to what we've been living with.

Established last year to stimulate the growth of prepaid group practices
through the private sector, Kaiser-Permanente Advisory Services is engaged in
discussions with Ford Motor Company and with General Motors and Chrysler
to study the feasibility of developing a community-wide prepaid group practice program in Detroit.

Another organization, the National Association of Employers on Health
Maintenance Organization (NAEHMO), was created in 1976 by the business
community in Minneapolis, which had previously done a remarkable job of
promoting HMO development in the twin cities of Minneapolis and St. Paul.
NAEHMO's objective is to assist its member companies—roughly 120 now—in
sponsoring and working with HMOs and in offering employees HMO membership as an alternative to traditional insurance coverage.

There are other indications of renewed business interest in HMOs. Individual success stories are gaining wide attention:[22] the closed-panel prepaid
group practice opened last year by R. J. Reynolds Industries for the company's
Winston-Salem, North Carolina, employees; the open panel IPA-HMOs in five
Wisconsin cities organized as a result of explorations begun nearly a decade
ago by Employers Insurance of Wausau, which continues to administer the
plans; and various other of the nation's 180 or so HMOs serving some 7 million
subscribers.

Insurance carriers, more than other industries, have tended to see HMO
sponsorship as a logical extension of their business. As of May 1977, 22
insurance companies were reported involved in 50 HMOs in 25 states; with
the "Blues" involved—as sponsor, administrator, or promoter and marke-
ter—in 107 HMOs.[22]

Proponents of industry involvement in establishing HMOs see the
approach as an avenue toward recreating a market in health services, as the
only viable alternative to increased government regulation. The HMO, in this
view, brings the entire system under control, so that it effectively begins to
regulate itself:

When you have your own HMO, you have your own utilization
review, your own quality control program, you own data system
built in. You have control of the costs and the services, you have a
communication vehicle with the beneficiaries of your health insur-
ance—in short, you have the whole ball of wax.

                                        Bynum E. Tudor

A similar line of reasoning was at the heart of the original health maintenance strategy enunciated in 1971 by Paul Ellwood and his staff. Ellwood is

still insistent that regulation is no answer, but he may be more open to variations short of fully developed HMOs than he once was:

> Where HMOs have been started, they have done extremely well. But these things are very difficult to start. It's a big deal, trying to radically restructure a $150 billion industry. There are serious barriers to HMOs and we have learned that many of the things we hoped to accomplish through HMOs can also be achieved through organizational arrangements that make fewer demands on the system. The HMO experience taught us that if we want to change the health system we have to come up with some way of doing it in stages.

Ellwood still holds to the principles undergirding the health maintenance strategy. The fundamental objective remains the hope of restoring a market in health services. The essential difference now is a heightned sense of urgency, on grounds that there may not be time to develop pure HMOs fast enough to achieve sufficient control over costs:

> We will have to be terribly creative, it seems to me, about coming up with schemes that go part way toward a real market and have built into them incentives to go further. And we are going to have to do it fast. Because I am under the impression that time really is running out on the market—that if market forces are going to play any significant role in the health system, they are going to have to be introduced immediately.

From the HMO experience, Ellwood extracts the essential conditions that he believes industry should bear in mind in adopting any cost containment scheme: It has to be comprehensive and deal with all aspects of the problem at once. Otherwise, holding down prices in one sector will simply lead to increases in another. It has to rely on the "big buttons" for success, not on piecemeal controls on one element at a time. The ideal way to pull the pieces together, Ellwood suggests, "is simply to have as the basic pricing unit the annual per capita costs in a community for individuals to get all the medical care they need."

If the objective is to restore the free market, then the approach ought to "restructure the circumstances under which people make their buying decisions." Thus, some cost-sharing for all but the poor ought to be instituted and comparative information on alternative sources of care ought to be disseminated. Consumers ought to have to commit themselves for a fairly extended period of time to where they will go for their health care, so that the circumstances in a health "crisis" will not be allowed to dominate and distort the choice. This implies that multispecialty groups are important because consumers do not know in advance what kind of providers they will need. It also suggests that employers ought to give employees a choice of where they will spend their health care benefit—almost like a voucher—and the relative costs of the different alternatives ought to be reflected in the price the purchaser pays. "In other words, health care consumers ought to be out shopping."

The provider side of the ledger is more complex, Ellwood believes, but as a start, providers ought to be aggregated into manageably sized groups (not necessarily HMOs) that allow calculations to be made of what their care is costing relative to comparable groups of providers:

> Without going to the big benefit package, without requiring risk sharing, without eliminating fee for service, and without requiring a group practice, it seems to me by aggregating physicians and then experience-rating them, you can create a device with the seeds of continuing change built into it which still has the capacity to contain costs.

The change begins to occur when the providers are aggregated for pricing purposes—even if in artificial groups—and begin working together in competition with other such groups. The competitive realities will encourage them to police their members or to exclude from membership those physicians in the area whose wasteful practice patterns inflate the costs of the group. Ellwood counsels businesses interested in changing the delivery system to enlist the support of the most prestigious sources of medical care in their community. He recommends that industries start their own delivery systems where possible, and concludes with a word of caution:

> I don't think you can expect to see instant returns. You won't immediately save money on market-oriented approaches any more than you will in a regulated system. What you are really hoping to do is to set in motion a series of steps that will ultimately change the shape of the curve of health care costs, bringing it back into line with the consumer price index for services generally.

In intermediate stages, and as variations on the HMO theme, there are several proposed models that may have cost-saving potential. The 1974 Conference Board report describes two examples.[23] One is a nonprofit occupational health clinic in Columbus, Indiana, serving the employees of Cummins Engine Company and, as of that writing, twelve other member firms, with another twenty waiting to join. The second is an HMO-type company health service organized by Gates Rubber Company in Denver, Colorado, which blends prepayment through a nonprofit financing arm with a multispecialty, fee-for-service in-house clinic providing both occupational and nonoccupational care. Similar opportunities exist elsewhere for smaller firms to contract for a wide range of occupational health services.[24]

A third model is being refined by Gilbeart Collings, the medical director of New York Telephone Company. Collings advocates a "health care management" approach, in which the industrial physician undertakes to develop with the employee a "lifetime health strategy" and then to help the employee procure from the external health system the services (periodic health assessments, preventive procedures, and treatment as indicated) implied in the overall strategy.[25] What this model seems to lack is the closed financing system to which the HMOs and fee-for-service practices with tight utilization review owe their cost control capability.

A fourth possible model is one we have hypothesized[26] and are currently exploring with several industries. It envisages "hybrid" industry-sponsored prepaid health plans meshing the firm's in-house clinical capacity with the external fee-for-service delivery system and the employee benefit package. The hybrid could be established by large, geographically concentrated industries acting alone or by smaller and more dispersed firms banding together. Like other prepaid health plans, it would offer subscribers—in this case employees and their families—a comprehensive range of prepaid health care as an alternative to traditional insurance coverage. Numerous potential problems in implementing the model have yet to be resolved but it seems to contain the essential elements of cost containment in health care: a closed system with a fixed budget and a defined population. Many other models can be developed, some perhaps more innovative, more fully developed, or promising than the ones touched on here. The challenge over the next several years will be not only to identify and disseminate word of seemingly effective innovations in personal health care being carried out by industry, but more important to set in motion a careful evaluation process. Organizers of new programs ought to be delineating their experiences as fully as possible, in quantitative and qualitative terms: What services are being provided to what population groups with what characteristics? How are the providers organized and interacting and to what extent have the new arrangements required them to deviate from their customary practices? What are they earning for the services they are providing? How are the different units of service (physician visits, hospital admissions, and lengths of stay) being financed, utilized, and monitored and what are they costing per person per year? Is there convincing evidence that the costs of the new program are different from the costs of the previous approach? What evidence is there that the care is of good quality (perhaps using as indices consumer satisfaction and measurable outcomes such as morbidity, mortality, and absenteeism).

An assessment such as this will provide an adequate basis for reaching sound conclusions. The virtue of "alternative delivery systems" is that they invite comparisons among possible delivery systems so that those that are proved most cost-effective and most satisfying to providers and patients can be identified and promoted.

Industry as Consumer: Health Planning and Consumer Health Information

From the dilemmas arising out of industry's expanded responsibilities as financer and provider of health care, it is a short step to a more active role in efforts at the community level to improve the delivery system and, at the level of individual decision-making, to assist workers in becoming better informed consumers of health care. Exploring piecemeal cost control strategies for employee benefit packages, or contracting with the external delivery system for supplementary services that may seem inadequate or inefficient can impress on industry the complexity of the problems in the health care delivery system, and the extent to which they are interlocking and self-perpetuating. These experiences have compelled some in industry to rephrase the question, shifting its focus from a limited perspective on how the firm can moderate the rising cost of its benefit package or rationalize its in-house services to a more global view of the delivery system as a whole and an attempt to discern why costs are rising throughout the system and what can be done.

When the focus moves to the community's health care services, a logical step for industry is to look for an active consumer role either in the federally and state-authorized health planning and regulatory process or through an expansion of the traditional functions of hospital trustees. Industry can also exert its influence as a consumer of health care on the state and national levels in the formulation of public policy bearing on health as well as in activities directed at the individual employees who are the ultimate health care consumers. Some employers are developing programs to encourage their employees to take batter care of themselves and to become informed and judicious users of health care services. Although these activities derive much of their impact from industry's involvement as a purchaser of care, they also can be viewed as constituting a consumer role for industry.

The concept of industry as a voice for the health care consumer is hardly new. Labor unions in the United States are widely recognized as the first organized and vocal consumers of health care, and business executives have long been a mainstay of hospital boards and voluntary health agencies. The difference now comes from the altered challenges and rewards. Where facility development and internal management may once have been a sufficiently broad focus, success in the future will hinge on quality of care in a setting of efficient and cost-effective regional health systems.

Community Health Planning

A consumer in official health planning parlance is quite simply a nonprovider, someone who holds no fiduciary position in the health care industry nor derives therefrom more than one-tenth of his or her gross annual income. Consumers have a defined and, on paper, substantial piece of the health planning action as most recently outlined in the National Health Planning and Resources Development Act of 1974 (P.L. 93-641). The instrumentalities through which the planning is to be conducted include 212 local health systems agencies (HSAs), covering the entire nation and, in each state, a state health planning and development agency, advised by a statewide health coordinating council (SHCC). It is in the HSAs and to a lesser extent the SHCCs that industry's influence is being felt. As the quotations in the box (see pp. 76–77) attest, opinion is divided on the potential of the HSAs, but it is too soon to judge them fairly. Structures are now being created and alliances forged. In some parts of the country industry is seeing in the fledging HSAs and SHCCs an opportunity to participate in decisions that could ultimately manifest themselves in the cost, quality, and scope of health care available to employees.

Because health planning is essentially a political process,[1,2] the HSAs have sought to recruit consumer members who can represent particular constituencies and thereby fortify the agency's power base and legitimacy. Business executives and labor leaders are seen by HSAs as representing important segments of the community to attract into the planning process, not only because of the constituencies (groups of employees or members) they represent, but also because of their purchasing power in the health market, the capital investment decisions they can often influence, and the technical expertise they can bring to the planning task.

Organized health planning has been accompanied by a subtle but important shift in the quid pro quo underlying industry's involvement in community-level health care enterprises. As hospital trustees, or board members for local Blue Cross Associations and other voluntary health organizations (heart, cancer, and lung associations, United Fund drives, and similar organizations of which there are some 25,000 in the United States), volunteers from industry brought prestige, social contacts, and the utility their names might provide for fund raising purposes. In exchange for their contributions they reaped enhanced prestige and the self-fulfillment that comes from community service. While wearing a trustee hat, they generally gave their loyalty to the institution or organization on whose board they were sitting and only inferentially to the broader community, less still to the industry from which they had come. This conventional relationship is now changing, largely to accommodate a new perception that the nation's resources for health care are limited and that objectives need to be redefined accordingly. One concrete expression of that growing perception can be found in the evolution of health planning.

In the period preceding World War II, "the golden years for medical philanthropy,"[3] advances in medicine and public health were stimulated almost exclusively by private voluntary contributions. After the war, the importance of private philanthropy in health began to be eroded by the rising tide of public financing and private insurance.

In 1946, Congress enacted the Hospital Survey and Construction (Hill-Burton) Act, providing federal subsidies for hospital construction, which had flagged seriously throughout the Depression and the war. To qualify for Hill-Burton funds, states were required to establish hospital planning units responsible for inventories of existing facilities and priorities for expansion. Frequently amended over the years, the original Hill-Burton Act has been called "one of the most advanced statements of public policy ever made in this country for the development of regionalized medical care."[4] That regionalization remains an elusive goal more than three decades later demonstrates an axiom of health policy: "a public policy pronouncement, however earnest its intent, is not be confused with a pragmatic achievement."[4]

A series of developments in the mid-1960s extended the boundaries and defined the structures of health planning and gave both momentum and direction to the planning process as it is now conceived. In 1963 the Hill-Harris amendments to the Hill-Burton Act authorized, in section 318, project grants for local nonprofit corporations charged with planning health facilities and governed by boards of community leaders and health providers.

For these local planning entities, Congress had found its models in as many as a dozen metropolitan regions where voluntary councils for planning health facilities had existed in some cases for twenty years and more. By the close of the 1960s, more than eighty areawide hospital planning agencies had been established[5] and some were expanding their horizons to permit a broader view of health services than only those delivered in hospitals.[6]

The Hill-Harris amendments were less than four years old when Congress replaced them with a more global piece of legislation, the Comprehensive Health Planning (CHP) and Public Health Services Amendments (P.L. 89-749),

HEALTH PLANNING: THE OPTIMISTS AND THE PESSIMISTS

Judith R. Lave: Health planning is in its infancy at the moment, and as you read the literature you find that people are either optimists or pessimists. The pessimists foresee the planners becoming supporters of the status quo. They point to the failure of regulation in other industries and suggest that the regulatory agencies tend to become captured by the organizations they were created to regulate. The optimists argue that no planning got us where we now are and planning can't make us any worse off.

Spencer C. Johnson: I worry about the prognosis for P.L. 93-641 but I do believe that it is the last opportunity we will have to maintain a pluralistic health system in this country. If health planning fails, we are going to have something very monolithic, a very rigid type of resource allocation and probably from the top down. My fear is that planning has come at the wrong time. The two enemies of the health planning movement—which is only about ten years old—are time and money. I believe it could work given time. But the social pressures for cost control, quality, and availability of medical services are so strong now that they threaten to overcome the health planning process before it is cleared up and moving.

Theodore E. Chester: I'm trying to be convinced here about the American way. But I wonder. Take my home town, Manchester, England. We have twenty hospitals there. The president of my university was a medical man who was not interested in any politics. He had told me that before the war there were at least twenty hospitals and they were all competing with one another as you are describing in your country. He decided to try to bring them together, as president of the university, and he invited them all to

supplemented the following year by the Partnership for Health Act (P.L. 90-174). Now health planning was to be comprehensive, taking account of developmental aspects of health services generally and health manpower, in addition to various types of health facilities. Elimination of needless duplication was to be an emphasis, along with conspicuous consumer participation in a "partnership for health" among federal, state, and local governments, providers, and consumers.

meetings at his house, and he got nowhere fast. He became a convinced supporter of what you call socialized medicine because he felt that this was the only way that anything could be achieved on a coordinated basis. What I fail to see is how you Americans are going to be able to do these things yourselves without the intervention of the government.

Richard M. Martin: I don't think the answer is in yet.

Chester: Then what can the answer be? You spend $140 billion and increase it every year by 14 percent. How long can you wait for the answer to come in?

Martin: But if we get enough people—maybe it is too much to expect—but if you get the private sector, this massive group out there that pays most of the bill. . . .

Chester: But the private sector does not speak with one voice. It's a very diverse entity.

Martin: That's right. But there are also diverse ways of going after the problems.

Chester: If your HSAs have no authority, as you suggest, then what you're saying is you have to educate people. How do you do this? Do people want to be educated? Can anybody educate other people without the delivery system's being changed?

R. K. deCamp: May I interject—I'm from the Pittsburgh HSA and I can't restrain myself any longer. I think that if what we mean by a monolith is some great federal takeover, then it's doomed to failure for the same reasons that the government can't close Navy yards, arsenals and Public Health Service hospitals. It is the private sector that is going to make it work or it will not work at all. We have the last shot, and it's the only shot in my view. I think it can work.

The CHP legislation set up a nationwide system for regionally based health planning by some 200 areawide "b" agencies (so called because created in section 314b of the act) and state-level "a" (for 314a) agencies. The CHP planning councils could be either public or nonprofit—the majority were the latter, with about half their funding from the federal grants provided for in the statute. B agencies were required to raise half their funds locally and often found health care providers most cognizant of their activities and willing to support them. This created a widespread impression that the b agencies were often in the fiscal pockets of providers and tended to undermine their credibility as regulators. The statute was sufficiently vague that resolution of ambiguities consumed some two to four years of organizational development efforts in most b agency areas. Health planning was only weakly linked to authority for decision-making. Having been granted no meaningful statutory authority by the CHP legislation, many of the agencies were slow or unable to find effective levers with which to move the system.

Meanwhile, the major lever through which health planning now exerts its influence—the certificate of need process—was developing in parallel. New York State led the way for "planning with teeth" by enacting the 1964 Metcalf-McClosky Act. This was the progenitor of state certificate of need laws, which prohibit important changes in health care facilities and services without a prior determination by a governmental agency that the change is justified by need. Grounded in theoretical and empirical observations signaling defects in the health care market, certificate of need spread gradually during the late 1960s and early 1970s and is now one of health planning's major functions, mandated by federal statute (P.L. 93-641). The theory holds that widespread third-party financing of health care has removed the financial responsibility for overexpansion from the hospital, which can simply pass on the costs in higher per diem rates paid by the general public through private insurance and tax-supported public financing programs. Unnecessary capital expenditures by hospitals (in the form of excess beds and a superabundance of high-technology equipment) are believed to fuel inflation throughout the health care system, not only driving up hospital rates per se, but also diverting investments that might otherwise have been spent on lower cost alternatives to hospital care, perhaps ambulatory and long-term care and home health services. Certificate of need laws were enacted by legislatures in about half the states in response to public pressure to contain rising health care costs, and particularly the cost of a hospital stay.

The upward trend in costs was already set before 1965, when it was accelerated by the explosion of public financing of health services resulting from Medicare and Medicaid. Directed specifically at enlarging access to care for the indigent (Medicaid) and the elderly (Medicare), both programs sought to remove inequities without altering the structure of the delivery system. To some extent, both have succeeded in that mission, but not without generating predictable cost escalation, in turn intensifying the government's efforts to bring costs into line. Congressional amendments in 1972 (Section 1122 of the Social Security Amendments) authorized states to make portions of federal reimbursement for Medicare, Medicaid, and Maternal and Child Health services contingent on state approval of capital expenditures.

Sieverts wrote in 1977 that "about 80 percent of the states have signed section 1122 agreements with the federal government, leaving only about four states at this writing that have neither a certificate of need law nor a section 1122 program."[7] Over time the certificate of need process has become increasingly sophisticated and involved,[8,9] as has its relationship to local and state health planning organizations, empowered, since the beginning of most state programs, to review and comment on certificate of need applications. Still the link between planning and decision-making was relatively weak and "by the early 1970s, the continuing rise in the cost of medical care, growing concern with the quality of care, and the emergence of national health insurance as a major policy issue, impelled attempts to design a more effective health planning system. These efforts resulted in the passage of P.L. 93-641."[10]

The health systems agencies (HSAs) now entrusted with the public mandate to establish goals and objectives and develop rational plans for the allocation of health care resources in the areas they serve are similar in most respects to the b agencies from which they issue. Sieverts finds various differences, two of which he calls "important," between the b agencies and the HSAs: first, "a marked narrowing of focus of areawide health planning in P.L. 93-641," embracing the health system and excluding environmental and other issues only tangentially related to the delivery of health care; second, intended funding levels substantially higher for HSAs than for CHPs, although to date, the funds allocated are well below the authorized levels. Both changes are clearly intended to strengthen health planners' hands. In addition, the act sought to give the HSAs authority in the allocation of federal grant monies and, through majority representation on the SHCCs, some opportunity to oversee the state government in its regulatory activities.[11]

Industry Involvement in Health Planning

Despite the strengthening refinements embodied in the latest generation of health planning, two fundamental weaknesses persist that offer industry a particular opportunity to influence the process. First, although the HSAs have more official authority than did their predecessors, health planning and the certificate of need process still lack an effective voice in third-party financing decisions, which largely determine how health services are organized and delivered. The planning process is still sufficiently diffuse that leverage will remain contingent on the power base the agency can build and the political clout it can command. And industry's potential clout, as a payer for care, is very substantial, and very much needed:

> The problem we have in health planning is the development of a constituency. The doctors have a constituency and a social fabric in this country. You say doctor and it calls to mind the golden age of medicine and so forth. You say hospital and you can trace that back too, and sanitarium, and sewage, and public health. You say planning and people stare at you. Say comprehensive health planning —who's going to go out on a rainy Wednesday night to go to a meeting about that?
>
> Spencer C. Johnson

Second, despite expectations that most HSAs will ultimately be funded more adequately than their CHP precursors, they will probably continue to experience difficulty attracting and holding a staff with technical expertise to match the providers they hope to regulate. Worse, delays in full funding of the planning act have made the transition from comprehensive health planning agency to HSA an austere one. According to Anthony T. Mott, Executive Director of the Finger Lakes HSA in Rochester, New York:

> HSAs are in very poor financial condition. Ever since the law was passed, I've been laying off people faster than I can count them. My staff of thirty has dwindled to fourteen and though we are still reasonably successful at getting deeply into the major capital expansion projects that come our way, realistically, we are pretty hard pressed to stay up with the long-range planning of many of the twenty-three hospitals in our region. We just don't have the resources.

Industry can help fill this gap by lending staff to the HSA and providing technical assistance, and, according to Richard Martin of Goodyear Tire & Rubber in Akron and president of the HSA there, through financial support which he views as an essential expression of the commitment needed from industry:

> If you're going to get involved with an HSA and make it work, you're not going to get by with the per capita allowance from the federal government. So what we did in Akron was to go to the corporate community and point out to them the irony of budgeting, nationally, a mere $125 million to plan for a $140 billion expenditure. If you can convince these corporate people that the HSA is viable, they understand return on investment. In spite of reductions in federal support last year, we were able to add staff to our HSA.

Martin calls for a full and unequivocal commitment, but lesser degrees of possible involvement can also be helpful to the HSA without being onerous to the firm. On a basic level, industry can demonstrate cooperation with the HSA by making employee benefits consonant with the goals articulated by the HSA, and by letting providers know that the firm will not pay—through employee benefits or through investments—for any projects lacking HSA approval. Banks, insurance companies, and bonding companies in particular can inadvertently frustrate the goals of cost containment and promote possibly injudicious expansion of costly health care facilities and services by bailing out hospitals in financial trouble.[1]

An illustration of industry cooperation with health planning is found in a recent agreement between Michigan Blue Cross–Blue Shield and Ford, General Motors, and Chrysler, which stipulates that providers will not be reimbursed for services involving expensive new equipment that has not been approved by the HSA.[2] With some $450 million currently invested in health-related facilities, the Equitable Life Assurance Society has established a policy of withholding all such investments in the future until the proposed project has been approved by the HSA. The company says, in a Washington Business Group on Health survey, that "we have tried to target our investments so as to increase the availability of ambulatory care, e.g., neighborhood health centers, and enhance the efficiency and effectiveness of community hospitals."[2]

On the intermediate level, industries can encourage their employees to participate in community health planning, can offer the financial and technical assistance that the agencies badly need, and can provide participating employees with orientation and training:

> *If the HSAs are to be successful, they will need informed boards. I believe this means that business and labor have a responsibility to make sure that their representatives to these boards have a good understanding of the problems. Evaluations have shown that consumer representatives to health planning boards have been largely ineffective because they have been unable to handle interactions with providers and have deferred to the providers as the experts. If business and labor are truly interested in influencing health planning, the first step is to be sure that their representatives in the process are armed with the facts they need to stand up to the providers.*
>
> Judith R. Lave

The third level of industry involvement in health planning is in a leadership role. There are several current examples of this role and historical precedents for it. As Anthony Mott points out:

> *P.L. 93-641 is new and HSAs are new, but health planning per se is not. It has been around on a voluntary basis for twenty or thirty years in a number of communities, chief among them Rochester, Pittsburgh, Cleveland, and Detroit. The motivation for the planning came from different directions in each city but it came very clearly in Rochester from the business and industrial sector's saying enough is enough.*

Mott attributes the early Rochester success to one man, Marion Folsome, a senior executive in Eastman Kodak who had enough influence in the banking community to stop the flow of money into recalcitrant health care institutions. Health planning in Rochester over the past two to three decades has held down the construction of hospital capacity and emphasized the development of alternatives to hospital care—neighborhood health centers, satellite clinics, home health care. Folsome left to serve as secretary of HEW and the late Joe Wilson of Xerox followed him for a time as Rochester's corporate health czar. The successful campaign to hold down the bed supply (Rochester has 3.5 beds per 1,000 population, compared with 4.5 nationwide) is credited in large measure for the low hospital use (629 days per 1,000) of Eastman Kodak employees in Rochester. By contrast, Kodak employees elsewhere average many more days in the hospital, 800 per 1,000 in Buffalo and Boston, 700 in

Cleveland, and 900 in Detroit. Rarely is the power Folsome could command concentrated in the hands of one individual, but one large industry in a small medical market or several working together in a larger one can have a similar impact. Goodyear Tire & Rubber in Akron, Ohio, has also been very effective in influencing the planning process.

As president of the HSA in Akron, member of the Ohio SHCC, and a Goodyear executive, Richard Martin has an unusual opportunity to marshal the resources of local industry in the health planning enterprise:

> There is almost no limit to what you can do in the HSA if you begin drawing on your company resources—financial people, people who understand the money market, industrial relations people who understand the operation and staffing of any enterprise, construction people who can help deal with architects and general contractors. The potential for hospitals to achieve savings in all these areas is substantial.

By tapping these various resources and interjecting them into the hospital planning process, Martin says, the Akron HSA has been able to streamline hospital planning to the point of averting some $20 million in costs the community would otherwise have absorbed over the next ten years. Described more fully elsewhere,[3,4,5] the Akron experience has come to be viewed as a bellwether for the role industry can have in community health planning. How widely that experience can be generalized remains to be seen as HSAs develop. Akron has an unusual concentration of corporate power for a city of its size (250,000), and that factor may be a critical ingredient in the Akron HSA's influence.

Other examples of industry participation in HSAs suggest that Akron is not unique. In Detroit, General Motors is a powerful force behind health planning[6] and Michigan Blue Cross–Blue Shield, together with Ford, GM, and Chrysler, has developed a comprehensive cost containment plan which includes provisions for close cooperation with community health planning.[7] Pittsburgh, Pennsylvania, has an ongoing tradition of active industry involvement in community health planning,[8,9] and a group of business executives in Portland, Maine, at the instigation of the HSA there, is currently developing an organization to work alongside the HSA.[10] Alcoa encourages employees in many of its locations to serve on HSA boards and financially supports local health planning through the Alcoa Foundation;[11] Employers Insurance of Wausau has been actively involved in health planning in Wisconsin.[12,13] Many other HSAs across the country are undoubtedly receiving valuable support from both management and labor components of industry.

Still, the performances of both industry and the HSAs in promoting cooperation have met with mixed reviews. Some HSAs have shunned industry participation, according to Mott, for reasons he fails to understand:

> There are many communities in the country where local businesses and industries have attempted to get involved in the HSAs and

have had the door slammed in their faces. From the HSAs' perspective, I can't imagine their thinking, but I know it has happened.

Martin wonders how hard industry tried:

> I hear large corporations say they can't get on an HSA board—can't get elected. These are successful companies that have been involved in the community yet they say they can't get onto a project review committee because it's a political group, or a provider-run group, and the door's closed. I'm a little dubious. All it takes to become involved is determination and a little effort to understand the health delivery system in the community. Collect the data and ask the questions and find out what's really going on. Pretty soon you'll be indispensable.

Mott's experience confirms that industry has sometimes been slow to take up the challenge, even in Rochester with its history of industrial leadership in health planning:

> I read about the corporate concern over rising health care costs and I wait for business representatives to begin beating down the door of the Rochester HSA looking for a piece of the action. But, I regret to say, it's just not happening. We certainly could make good use of the expertise, ability, muscle, and voice that the corporate sector could bring to this process.

Aside from the issue of health care costs, private industry should, in theory, find several good reasons to support local health planning. Philosophically, there is the appeal the private sector ought to find in the local autonomy and private initiative encouraged through HSAs:

> Goodyear supports viable HSAs that have a goal to benefit the total community, even though they're a form of regulation. We support them because the regulatory decisions are made on the local level where we feel they belong.
>
> Richard M. Martin

As a practical matter, local decision-making should enable industry, in planning a corporate expansion or relocation, to have a hand in designing a health system to meet the needs of employees. From an industrial relations standpoint, health planning may be that rare arena in which management and labor can work together toward common goals.

Finally, the cost imperative is inescapable—particularly the problem of hospital costs. Hospital cost escalation is largely a function of excess capacity and overcapitalization. The problem of excess hospital beds has been studied in considerable detail.[14] In a recent report to HEW, Walter McClure of Inter-Study concluded that without deleterious effects on health, hospital capacity in the United States could be reduced by at least 20 percent—"if done appropriately and in an orderly manner."[15] McClure adduces evidence of the need to reduce hospital capacity from fifteen years of research showing that "beds beget patients," driving up utilization rates, and conversely that reduction in hospital bed capacity reduces use. In short, "hospital use is correlated with hospital capacity rather than with indices of health or need."[15]

A reduction of capacity must, however, be accomplished carefully to achieve maximal savings which, McClure predicts, would be dissipated in increased labor and capital intensity of the existing beds without effective restraints. McClure's calculations demonstrate that much greater cost savings are realizable through the more sensitive and difficult process of closing down major elements—hospital wings, clinical services, or whole hospitals—than by merely reducing the bed complement in many facilities. The problem of excess hospital beds, in McClure's view, is fundamentally a socio-political rather than a technical challenge and is likely to be solved only if "the public and providers can be educated to accept some trade-off between the more lavish level of hospital care to which they have become accustomed and their desires to free resources for other purposes more productive of health and well-being."[16]

This observation points to industry—both in the payer role where the employee benefit package has helped to shape the public taste for "lavish" care and in the consumer role, where industry's tradition of involvement on hospital boards confers an opportunity and perhaps a responsibility for industry to lead the way to a fundamental redirection of the priorities motivating hospital administrations.

As we have seen, expenditures for hospitalization are a prime target for cost control. Hospital costs account for almost 40 percent of the nation's health care expenditures and hospital charges are rising faster than other health care prices (a 13 percent increase from 1974 to 1975, compared with 9.9 percent for medical care generally, 11.8 and 7.8 for physicians' and dentists' fees, and 7.4 for drugs).[17] Economic factors (virtually inexhaustible demand, a flawed incentive system, and the third-party payment scheme which pays about 90 percent of hospital expenditures) have fueled this inflation, along with closely related social and political factors of which industry is showing increased awareness.

In the past, hospital trustees have seldom exercised the full measure of authority they officially possess. Hospitals have been governed through an informal system of checks and balances in which the physician staff controls the medical decisions, leaving nonmedical aspects of the hospital's operation to the administrative staff. This system of "dual control," Anne and Herman Somers argue, "often means no control."[18] Sometimes it has meant that the medical and administrative staffs have neutralized each other. More often, however, the administration has defined its mission to coincide with the wishes of the medical staff, knowing that the institution's quality and viability depend on its capacity to attract and hold a first-rate medical staff.

Since the highest professional prestige in medicine is associated with specialized technological care, the administrator's rule of thumb is to keep his institution well-appointed and equipped with the latest in technological advances, based on the belief that it probably will pay off in improved patient care. Since the cost of these investments can be passed on to third parties without noticeably burdening the patient, all the incentives have pointed to continuous upgrading and expansion of the facility and its equipment:

> *I don't think there are villains in the system—grabby physicians or ineffectual hospital administrators. By and large people are responding to the sets of incentives they see in front of them.*
> Judith R. Lave

The incentives to tailor the hospital to the physician's specifications are largely a product of the historical view of the hospital as "the doctor's work-shop"[18]—a place where he could bring his private patients without assuming administrative or financial responsibilities. The fact that physicians can and often do have admitting privileges at more than one hospital liberates them still further from accountability to a particular institution. The hospital, on the other hand, very much needs the physicians if it is to compete successfully for patients and remain solvent.

This traditional arrangement, the Somers recently argued, "long ago became an anachronism." But "only slowly are we coming to think of the hospital as being there primarily to serve patients rather than physicians."[18] With a gradual reformulation of the hospital's primary mission, a concurrent shift in the trustees' role will be required.

Historically, the function of trustees was to ratify the requests of the medical staff, articulate them to the community, and help raise the requisite funds to fulfill them. Consonant with the medical mystique that pervaded the community, this posture reflected the assumption that hospitals, as public charities, need not hew to the standards of efficient operation demanded in the marketplace for the private sector businesses which many of the trustees represented.

The looser standard for hospitals became difficult to justify from the perspective of the company absorbing a growing share of the extra costs that were generated. Business executives sitting on hospital boards began to feel conflicting pressures—from their corporations they sensed alarm over rising hospital costs and a desire to pull in the reins, yet the hospital's incentive system still called for relatively unconditional growth and expansion. Some of the companies, seeing in their representatives on hospital boards an opportunity to influence the investment decisions being made by the hospitals, initiated educational programs designed to equip their executives to bring the company's perspective on the need for medical care cost control into the hospital boardroom:

> *If you have the responsibility within a company for the costs of employee health care, it quickly becomes clear that you had better educate those people who are sitting on hospital boards. You'd better convince them that we simply cannot afford to give the doctors everything they say they need. You'd better impress on*

them the implications of letting the doctors purchase a $400,000 linear accelerator that won't be fully utilized because there's an underused Cobalt 60 in the next room and a betatron across the street. You'd better persuade them that it is in the interest of the community, and ultimately of the institutions they are serving, to say no to an unneeded investment, to say yes, we can do a better financial job of running this hospital.

Richard M. Martín

In the two dimensions Martin alludes to—internal management of the hospital and coordination with neighboring facilities—trustees' roles are expanding. Within the hospital, trustees have a responsibility to weigh the requests of the providers against the possible long-range costs and health benefits, to mediate conflicts between the medical and administrative staffs, and to set a tone that fosters cost consciousness throughout the institution. Some specific techniques are recommended by three University of Michigan researchers in a report published in the *Harvard Business Review*[19] and later expanded into a book.[20] The authors argue that "if every trustee in every hospital in the United States judged every expenditure request in terms of one question, 'What will happen to the health of my community if I say no?' and then said no whenever the answer was 'nobody knows,' or 'nothing,' or 'not much,' health care costs would drop precipitously."[19]

Within the broader community, the challenges and the potential for savings may be even greater. Merging and consolidating redundant facilities or services will, as McClure points out, be a long-haul process fraught with conflict. Loyalties to hospitals run deep among their various constituents— board members and local politicians who see the institution as a community asset, medical staffs and other employees for whom it represents financial stability, patients who prefer the convenience and security embodied in a nearby full-service hospital over some abstract ideal called a regionalized health system.

Alcoa's experience, reported to the Washington Business Group on Health, bears witness to the difficulties involved in bringing two hospitals together. In sixteen locations where Alcoa has plants, nineteen executives are serving on hospital boards, four as presidents. The consolidation of two community hospitals on the West Coast was said to involve a four-year effort on the part of an Alcoa plant manager who was instrumental in the process. Over fifty meetings were involved, some as far as a hundred miles away. The manager of an Alcoa plant in the Midwest has been working for over five years to bring about a merger, as yet unaccomplished, between two overlapping community hospitals. Alcoa has developed a training program for employees approached to become hospital trustees, in recognition, the company says, of "the importance of having responsible people serve on hospital boards."[21]

Education of executives is a major ingredient in industry's more active consumer involvement in hospital and local health planning. A separate but conceptually related activity being initiated by some companies is the broad-scale education of employees with the goal of promoting healthful lifestyles and of reducing wasteful use of health care services. These activities cut across all of industry's roles—as payer seeking to develop informed users of health benefits, as provider seeking to find mechanisms, such as elimination of hazards and toxins from the workplace, for successful primary prevention of disease, and as an informed consumer.

Individual Decisions about Health and Health Care

Within the past four years, the prevention of underlying causes of disease has emerged as a major emphasis in national health policy. It began with strong public statements, issued first by the Canadian then by the United States government, calling for a reexamination of the relationship between health and medical care.

The Canadian document, commonly referred to as the Lalonde report for the minister of national health and welfare under whom it was prepared, was a concise and articulate public sector reassessment of the priorities dictating national investments in health care.[1] On the basis of conventional mortality and longevity statistics, the report calculated the years of life lost by cause of death. The calculation revealed that the five most important causes of early death, in order, were motor vehicle accidents, ischemic heart disease, all other accidents, respiratory diseases and lung cancer, and suicide. Noting that "self-imposed risks and the environment are the principal or important underlying factors in each of the five major causes of death between age one and age seventy," the report concluded that "unless the environment is changed and the self-imposed risks are reduced, the death rates will not be significantly improved."[2]

The United States Public Health Service, in its June 1975 *Forward Plan for Health,* made similar observations about the root causes of death and disability and drew parallel conclusions.[3] Failing a dramatic scientific break-through, the United States government predicted, further expansion of the nation's health care system is likely to produce only marginal increments in health status. The best hope of real progress against untimely death and chronic disabling illness, it was argued, may lie instead in primary preventive strategies.

The term *primary prevention* encompasses interventions directed at eliminating exposure or susceptibility to agents of disease or injury rather than at detecting or repairing damage already done. Early detection and treatment of disease in order to change its course or outcome is customarily called *secondary prevention,* and activities directed at mitigating disability and dependence resulting from chronic diseases are sometimes referred to as *tertiary prevention.*[4] Primary prevention can be further broken down into activities seeking to identify potential agents of disease or injury and to remove them from the environment, on the one hand, and strategies to protect the individual who is exposed on the other. In the second instance, it is usually necessary to win the individual's cooperation and participation either once (for example to submit to an inoculation) or in an ongoing way (for example, to wear protective goggles or seatbelts, to give up cigarette smoking, or to take up exercising). Participation is often a problem also in secondary and tertiary prevention: the medical profession continues to search for good ways to achieve long-term patient compliance with therapeutic regimes such as medication to control hypertension.[5,6] But the issue of cooperation is nowhere more challenging than in health education where individuals need to be persuaded to alter their styles of life in order to avoid negative health consequences that may or may not result sometime in the relatively distant future.

Industry's perspective on health education is shaped by three main factors. One is the cost of health care. From the point of view of a payer for care, there is significance in the growing concensus in the health field that medical care may be reaching the limits of its ability to greatly affect the overall health status of the population. From this belief it may seem to follow that primary prevention could harbor long-range potential for real impact on health status and perhaps ultimately the cost of employee health benefits. The difficulty with this formulation is its assumption of a close relationship between health status and the cost of employee health benefits. The link may be tenuous; indeed, much of the "health care" covered in the benefit package may be discretionary use of procedures and services with little or no demonstrable impact on health. This is a possibility we discuss more fully in our look to the future (chapter 6).

Another factor is the time horizon. The payoffs that may be possible through health education and prevention are not yet calculable, nor are they likely to appear in the immediate future. As a result, the government tends to assign prevention a relatively low priority while channeling resources and attention into approaches with greater visibility and more chance of an immediate impact. Finally, there are political realities. For a democratic government to interject itself into its citizens' personal decisions as to how they will live their lives is a delicate business, with the spectre of coercion always close at hand:

> Speaking as one who occasionally has a drink or likes to drive a car fast sometimes, I feel adamantly that the first time you try to change my lifestyle through sanctions—whether through economic or political leverage—you've begun to move from a free to a coercive government and I will fight you all the way.
>
> Kenneth A. Platt

The case can be made that a society cannot afford to make health care a "right," as the United States has effectively done, without conditioning that right with a measure of individual responsibility. A strong spokesman for that case is John H. Knowles, president of the Rockefeller Foundation, who argues: "One man's freedom in health is another man's shackle in taxes and insurance premiums. I believe the idea of a 'right' to health should be replaced by the idea of an individual moral obligation to preserve one's own health—a public duty if you will."[7] But the philosophical argument, however compelling, does not negate the political sensitivity of the lifestyle issue. And so the government has always looked to the private sector for leadership and support in health education.

In fact, the private sector—and industry per se—has been a decisive force in health education since the president's 1971 health message to Congress called for new approaches and stimulated the creation of a President's Committee on Health Education. Stressing voluntary leadership in the private sector, the charge to the committee was to find "ways to develop in the general public a sense of 'health consumer citizenship.'" The President's Committee was chaired first by Joe Wilson of Xerox Corporation and then by R. Heath Larry of United States Steel Corporation. It delivered its final report to the White House in 1973, and recommended the formation of a National Center for Health Education, to be based in the private sector but with substantial federal support. The government's Center for Disease Control contracted with the private-sector National Health Council to study the feasibility of the proposed national center. And during the course of the feasibility study, enough interest and momentum developed in the private sector to stimulate the creation of the proposed National Center for Health Education, even before federal funding was assured. The National Health Council came out strongly in favor of the proposed center and it opened October 1, 1975.[8]

The federal government has since followed suit. Last year Congress enacted the National Consumer Health Education and Health Promotion Act of 1976, (P.L. 94-317), which provides for a national program of "health information, health promotion, preventive health services, and education in the appropriate use of health care," and establishes an Office of Health Information and Health promotion within HEW.

It is important to recognize that the elevation of health education to the status of a national priority is an endorsement only of the concept that the population appears to need better or more persuasive information on which to base decisions bearing on health and the use of health care services. It does not reflect evidence—as yet unavailable—that health education is an effective means of disseminating that information or of getting results:

> *People talk about prevention as if we knew how to do it, but we don't. It's a grossly underfunded and underexplored area. Prevention is just emerging from the Dark Ages.*
>
> Gilbeart H. Collings

The process of bringing health promotion into a more enlightened era has only begun. A long research agenda remains to be addressed.[9,10,11] Industry, in turn, will be challenged over the next several years to define the role that it will play:

> *Health education places particular strains on corporate policy. For most corporations, the concept of educating and influencing employees about how they live is a nontraditional role. And that raises all kinds of new issues and problems and threats to the traditional structure of corporate management-employee relationships. The question then arises, are the risks warranted? I believe they are. It is just ludicrous to think that the population—you and I—cannot improve our capacity to take care of ourselves, to influence our own health status, to be better spenders of our health benefits, to waste fewer dollars. And we will all be better off for it.*
>
> Willis B. Goldbeck

Summing Up

On concluding its year-long study of rising health care costs, the President's Council on Wage and Price Stability issued a strong challenge to the private sector:

> The American people generally are becoming increasingly unwilling to devote an ever larger portion of their personal income to health care. Although the full extent of the cost escalation has been somewhat hidden through the mechanism of third-party payments, taxes, payroll deductions, and direct employer and union payments to insurers, the day is coming, and coming fast we were told, when the people are going to discover how much they must increasingly sacrifice simply in order to maintain the status quo in health care services. When that day comes, we believe the people of this country will turn to the federal government and demand that it solve the problem. . . . Absent any major changes in the structure of the medical care system between now and then, the federal government will step in, and when that happens, we are going to be faced with a permanent problem which will defy solution. This does not have to happen. We are convinced

that an alternative to federal control of the health care system is available if promptly seized. . . . That alternative is a concerted and united effort on the part of industry and labor to control costs. . . . But make no mistake about it, the private sector must step up its efforts manyfold; it must apply the full measure of ingenuity and management skills which are so characteristic of the American system.[1]

In this first issue of the Springer Series on Industry and Health Care, we have seen that industry—both management and labor—plays a multidimensional and complex role in health care, with rising costs a precipitating factor and with concern for quality, equity, and access also very much in mind. As we have traced industry's involvement in health care, as payer, provider, and consumer, six broad challenges have emerged.

(1) *The benefit package* itself is at the core of the problem in an intimate but as yet inadequately understood relationship with rising costs. It seems clear that the extensive employer financing of health insurance has tended to blunt consumer consciousness of the costs of care, to permit the health care industry to constantly refine and expand its "product" (the mix, level and technological intensity of services provided), and to raise consumer expectations. The problem, now, is that the incremental building to the present level of expectations is a virtually irreversible process. Some soul searching may be needed by both labor and management if the cost problem is to be solved. That is the first challenge.

(2) *Cost containment activities* are being tried by industry in a variety of forms and settings and under various auspices. Considerable ingenuity is manifest in many of these efforts and some appear promising, although few have produced irrefutable evidence of effectiveness. Little is known about overlapping effects the various strategies may have nor about their possible unintended side effects both within the health system and beyond. For example, the gains in system-wide efficiency of closing down a community hospital may be lost in unemployment. Most of the cost containment strategies developed to date have ardent supporters and equally convinced detractors. And most appear to either require a major commitment of time and energy, which will have to be sustained over a period of years before results can reasonably be expected, or else to promise a quick but relatively minor payoff. The challenge will be to sort through these various possibilities, identify the ones that are best suited to local circumstances, and arrive at a comprehensive and well thought out approach that makes the most sense for the particular firm or union, for its employees or rank and file, and for the broader community of which it is a member.

(3) *Occupational health and safety* presents challenges as never before. Heightened awareness of the presence of environmental toxins and carcinogens in the workplace and the standard-setting activities of the Occupational Safety and Health Administration have already brought dramatic changes to the industries using dangerous substances in their production processes. A long-standing source of conflict, the employer's responsibility for workers' health and safety is being extended, and the occupational medical profession—

itself beset by conflicts and a crisis of accountability—is seeking to meet the new challenge. The Occupational Safety and Health Act purports to internalize within the firm the costs of preventing occupational disease and injury, but the long latency periods and insidious onset of most occupational disease, coupled with the mobility of the American work force, complicates the issue of employer responsibility. And the laudable goal of prevention is elusive in actual practice. Industries will have to come to grips with the proper and legal scope of their responsibilities for their workers' health and will then have to find the most effective and cost-efficient mechanisms through which to discharge this responsibility. Smaller and geographically more dispersed firms and industries will probably need to find creative ways of pooling their resources in order to meet their new obligations.

(4) *The market in health services* is seriously flawed and the government's response has been and will doubtless continue to be tightened regulation. Many analysts of the system look at rising costs and deduce that the nation is now poised at a crossroads, one path leading to more and tighter regulation and ultimately a monolithic nationalized health system; the other to a market-oriented pluralistic system with informed consumers choosing from among a range of alternative delivery systems. Those who favor the market approach are looking to industry for allies. Without this alliance, they see no other way to effect the needed changes and develop the alternative systems fast enough to avert an irretrievable decision to go down the regulatory path.

(5) *Health planning* at the community and state levels is a new and struggling discipline with a strong federal mandate and a large job to do. It opens opportunities for industry to influence the allocation of local resources for health care. It also badly needs industry's participation for the technical expertise, fiscal resources, and political leverage it can bring to the process.

(6) *Lifestyle* has been identified as an important contributor to premature mortality and chronic disability. Alcohol, cigarettes, motor vehicles, obesity, firearms, and stress contribute importantly to or actually cause many of the deaths and disabling injuries or diseases that occur among the young and middle-aged populations in our society. For this reason, new attention is being paid in public health circles to health education and promotion of healthful styles of living. Since many Americans spend most of their waking hours on the job, the workplace is a logical locus for implementing health promotion strategies. Very little is currently known, however, about how to persuade people to change their ingrained habits and any efforts to do so must tread lightly and conscientiously avoid violating the individual's civil liberties. Still, something ought to be done and industry clearly is in a position to take a leadership role. This is the last of the six central challenges.

In closing, there are two important dimensions to the problem of rising health care costs that have not been explored in this monograph but deserve mention. First, it is a nearly universal problem throughout the developed world. As we in this country search for solutions, we should not fail to look elsewhere for lessons—both positive and negative—and for a broader perspective. In her presentation at the Cornell Conference, Judith Lave cited data showing that health care costs have been rising more rapidly in several foreign countries than in the United States and observed:

> *Whereas we are naturally going to develop our strategies in the American context, we would do well to bear in mind that there is something going on here that doesn't necessarily have to do with a set of American institutions.*

Not only is there potential applicability to other nations of whatever solutions Americans can develop, but also much of value to be learned from international experiences, irrespective of disparities in the political, economic, social, and cultural milieus within which the various health systems operate.

Second, there is a demographic imperative that is contributing to rising health care costs. The work force is shrinking in relation to the proportion of dependent people in the United States population. The population is aging, and the twin causes are increases in life expectancy at birth and sustained reduction in fertility.[2] The proportion of people aged 65 and older has increased importantly since 1900 (from 4 percent to 10 percent in 1970),[3] and the oldest, and therefore least healthy, segment of the elderly population is growing fastest.[4] Of those 65 and older in 1930, 20 percent were 75 and older; by 1970 that percentage had risen to 38.[3] Those 85 and older were 5.7 percent of the 65 and older population in 1960, 6.7 percent by 1970, with 7.6 percent or 1.8 million Americans aged 85 and older forecast for 1980.[4] Comparing the utilization of health services among different age groups shows that the elderly use more services, and especially more inpatient services which fall on the high end of the cost spectrum. For example, 1973 hospital days per 1,000 population were, respectively, 898 for ages 15–44, 1698 for ages 45–64, and 4228 for ages 65 and above. Average lengths of hospital stay progressed from 5.7 days to 9.1 to 12.1, and physician visits per person per year, respectively, from 5 to 5.5 to 6.5.[4] The growing elderly population needs and receives more health care services.

This, then, is the broad context in which industry is confronting the challenge of rising health care costs in an era of limited resources. Future issues of the Springer Series will home in on discrete aspects of industry's involvement in the health care system. Here we hope we have shown that the potential impact industry can have if creatively and actively involved is great, mechanisms for involvement are available, and the need for creativity is palpable and pressing.

Issues for the Future

This last chapter should be viewed in a different light from the preceeding five. Our intention here is to be provocative, to polarize the issues, and to propose a conceptual matrix for industry's future discussions of health policy. Among the many health policy issues embedded in this monograph, we have identified two that appear to have particular relevance to the problem of health care cost control, and cost is the preeminent health concern of the day.

Rationing of Health Services

Everywhere we see evidence of rationing health services. States are unable to fully fund Medicaid programs, thus denying service to the poor. Health planning agencies turn down the petitions of community hospitals proposing to expand their capabilities. And a cap is put on hospital costs, thereby forcing hospitals to curtail services.

It is not illogical for society to establish procedures whereby scarce items are rationed, if necessary, to ensure that the disadvantaged received a basic share of the necessities of life, even if they are unable to pay for them. Adequate housing, food, and clothing, as well as a chance at a job that can help an individual realize his potential would be accepted by most citizens as rights in our culture. Health care is increasingly viewed as a right. What is odd about health services is the seeming presumption by policymakers that *all* components of medical services are of *equal value* and are essential. There has been little discussion about a truly basic "floor" consisting of health services that are considered a right for all individuals. Once identified, these services would be the focus of efforts to equalize access and would not be subject to coinsurance, deductibles, or other disincentives:

> In all systems, however "socialized," there is a certain free sector. The Germans, with 95 percent of the population publicly insured, still have quite a flourishing private health insurance system that is doing very well because it provides supplementary insurance for those who want it. And some people like to have a little bit more: they drink, or smoke tobacco, or would like to have a private room. Well, let them have it—why not? I do not believe that we should have a system which imposes a ceiling on everybody. What I do believe, very firmly, is that modern society, to be viable and peaceful, needs a floor below which no human being should fall.
>
> Theodore E. Chester

The floor would be set to assure access to such things as vaccination procedures, surgery for acute bleeding, and appropriate medical treatment for congestive heart failure. What is little discussed is that there is a large domain of medical services that are not of *clearly* demonstrated value, but are utilized by health professionals and subscribed to by their patients, the public. Why should it any more be the right of all individuals to be provided with available, but "unproved" or "optional" components of health care than to be furnished any other desired but not necessary item (spacious housing, gourmet food, or expensive clothing)?

Of course, it would be ideal if society could assure a standard of living at the highest level for all its members. The problem is that there are never enough consumer goods to fulfill all desires, and a government that begins allocating the nonessential ones is quickly drawn into setting priorities and making trade-offs. But the more deeply the government becomes involved in these complicated decisions, the further removed it is from a reliable index of whether the choices it is making are truly reflective of those that individuals in society would make if given the opportunity and adequate information.

This is precisely the problem that the concept of a right to health care has engendered. To the extent that a significant portion of medical services are "consumer items" that are not absolutely essential, why should they not be regarded in the same light as other desirable but not vital items? The critical missing concept in this context has been that of a floor of medical services below which no individual can go, and which is readily available to all, and of high quality.

If, as has repeatedly been emphasized in recent writings,[1,2,3,4] the availability and quantity of medical services can no longer be correlated with health status, the stage is set for a completely different analysis of our medical care system than the usual. Above the floor of necessary medical care, there is a group of "desirable but nonessential" services that can be provided to the disadvantaged by society if it wishes, similar to other social policies that seek some measure of income redistribution. And there will then remain a broad band of medical services that are optional consumer items, sometimes even of a luxury sort, such as elaborately furnished hospital rooms and special health professional coverage entirely on a convenience basis.

If we accept the concept of a floor for health services, then the companion question is whether we must establish a ceiling at the other extreme. The principal reason the country is experiencing so much agony on health care costs is the currently unchallenged assumption that all medical services are equally necessary, from which it follows that all medical care and associated costs fit without distinction into the same benefit package. What if the floor were established as a *minimum* benefit package, to which everyone is entitled? If "desirable" and "optional" medical services were bought in an open market with adequate information on prices and experiences, there would be no need for a ceiling, because then the purchase of these medical services could vie with other consumer items in terms of attractiveness to the consumer.[5]

It is apparent that if we were to establish a minimum benefit floor of medical services, and not worry about a ceiling on either individual or aggregate costs of medical services that are not absolutely essential, we would have a very different framework within which to consider questions of equity, access, and the financing of medical care. The alternative to this approach is to persist in regarding almost all medical services as essential and part of third-party financed benefits packages, and to continue with the elaboration and application of new technology irrespective of any proven effect on the health of patients. The results of this reactive posture will be steadily mounting costs for health benefit packages and increasing government regulation, coupled with complicated and imprecise rationing procedures, concerning which little intense and creative thinking has occurred.

Who Should Manage the System?

The second critical issue needing to be debated over the next several years is who can most cost-effectively manage the delivery of health services. Just as it will be necessary to come to grips with the issue of rationing, either by the floor-ceiling concept or by one which accepts all medical services as essential, so too must we decide whether the private sector shall continue to be entrusted with the running of the medical care apparatus for at least the next several years. The alternative would be for the government to be given the assignment of managing the nation's health services as it now runs the huge Veterans Administration and Department of Defense health systems. The present situation falls somewhere between two extremes, with the private sector still managing the health system but under increasing constraints imposed by governmental regulation. The decision for the future is whether to pursue more government or less government in health services.

In our view, a government-run health system is not the best answer; there is too much evidence that programs run from the top down fail to run smoothly and efficiently; evidence from other countries suggests that this observation holds for national health services. It does seem clear that if the private sector is to take the lead, it has a very limited time—because of the pressures of rising health care costs—to make the major changes that are needed in order to reestablish a functioning market in health services. These include providing information about health services to the public and establishing competitive alternative delivery systems. Informational barriers are falling in all the professions—including the medical profession—and it is a safe prediction that information about fees, practice experience, and clinical results achieved by individual physicians may well be available to the consuming public in the near future. Barriers to the development of delivery systems, such as prepaid health plans, which can serve as alternatives to solo practice, fee-for-service medicine, must be identified and removed. Incentives must be structured into reimbursement systems that maximize the involvement of physicians and all other providers in achieving the goal of cost-effective delivery of care. Informed consumers making active choices, based at least in part on considerations of cost, are an essential part of such an incentive system.

The concept of a floor for health services, accompanied by a wide range of discretionary services available for those who wish to purchase them, could lead over time to a situation where nonessential medical services are publicized in the media through appropriate and informative advertising and are thus given an opportunity—and a necessity—of proving themselves in a modified open market. The value of this approach is that it builds in self-correcting properties.

It seems unlikely that the private sector will be able to bring health care costs into line without confronting these two fundamental questions: can we agree on a minimum floor of health services that we can afford to subsidize for all who need them, and, above that floor, can we create a modified market in health services to facilitate expressions of personal preference? If we cannot achieve those two goals, then there will be no other option than for the government to expand its regulatory activities and ration health care.

Appendix

Conference Participants Quoted

Cornell University, Health Program for Business Executives
"Strategies for Controlling Medical Care Costs"
Ithaca, New York: May 5–6, 1977
and
Boston University Health Policy Institute
"Industry-Sponsored Health Programs"
Boston: June 3–4, 1977

Roger M. Battistella, Ph.D., Professor, Medical Care Organization, Cornell University, (May 5–6).

John J. Boardman, Jr., Executive Vice President, Kaiser-Permanente Advisory Services, Oakland, California, (May 5–6).

Douglas R. Brown, Ph.D., Director, Health Program for Business Executives, Cornell University, (May 5–6).

Thomas E. Burns, Consultant, Employee Compensation and Benefits, Corporate Employee Relations, General Electric Corporate Headquarters, Fairfield, Connecticut, (May 5–6).

Rick J. Carlson, J.D., Mill Valley, California, (June 3–4).

Theodore E. Chester, Professor, Dr. Jur., M.A., University of Manchester, England, (May 5–6).

Gilbeart H. Collings, M.D., General Medical Director, New York Telephone Company, New York, (May 5–6 and June 3–4).

R. K. deCamp, Associate Director, Health Systems Agency of Southwestern Pennsylvania, Pittsburgh, Pennsylvania, (May 5–6).

Stanley P. deLisser, EHE Health Services, Inc., New York, New York (June 3–4).

Paul M. Ellwood, Jr., M.D., President, Interstudy, Minneapolis, (May 5–6).

Willis B. Goldbeck, Executive Director, Washington Business Group on Health, Washington, D.C. (May 5–6 and June 3–4).

Timothy M. Harrington, Director of Research and Development, Blue Cross–Blue Shield of Massachusetts, Boston, (May 5–6).

Thomas Herriman, Amalgamated Clothing & Textile Workers Union, New York, (June 3–4).

Spencer C. Johnson, Professional Staff Member, Senate Human Resources Committee, Washington, D.C., (May 5–6).

Michael B. Jones, Partner, New York Office, Hewitt Associates, (May 5–6).

James E. Lapping, Director, Safety and Occupational Health, Building and Construction Trades Department, AFL–CIO, Washington, D.C. (June 3–4).

Judith R. Lave, Ph.D., Associate Professor of Economics and Urban Affairs, Carnegie-Mellon University, Pittsburgh, Pennsylvania (May 5–6).

Richard M. Martin, Manager, Health Services, Industry Relations, Goodyear Tire & Rubber Company, Akron, Ohio, (May 5–6 and June 3–4).

Eugene McCarthy, M.D., Department of Public Health, Cornell University Medical College, New York City, (May 5–6).

David F. McIntyre, Manager of Employee Benefits, General Mills, Minneapolis, (May 5–6).

Joseph M. Miller, M.D., Medical Care Associates, Inc., Boston, (June 3–4).

Anthony T. Mott, Executive Director, Finger Lakes Health Systems Agency, Rochester, New York, (May 5–6).

Kenneth A. Platt, M.D., Medical Director, Westminister Medical Clinic, Denver, (May 5–6).

Harold Richmond, M.D., Columbus Occupational Health Association, Columbus, Indiana, (June 3–4).

Jacob J. Spies, Assistant Vice President, Employers Insurance of Wausau, Wausau, Wisconsin, (May 5–6 and June 3–4).

Kevin Stokeld, Manager, Group Claims Department, Deere & Company, Moline, Illinois, (May 5–6).

C. Stephen Tsorvas, Consultant, Employee Benefits, General Electric Company, Fairfield, Connecticut, (June 3–4).

Bynum E. Tudor, Director, Corporate Employee Benefits, R. J. Reynolds Industries, Inc., Winston-Salem, North Carolina, (June 3–4).

Leon J. Warshaw, M.D., Vice President and Corporate Medical Director, Equitable Life Assurance Society of the United States, New York, (June 3–4).

Victor M. Zink, Director of Employee Benefits and Services, Industrial Relations Staff, General Motors Corporation, Detroit, Michigan, (June 3–4).

Notes

Chapter 1. Introduction

1. Executive Office of the President, Council on Wage and Price Stability: *The Complex Puzzle of Rising Health Care Costs: Can the Private Sector Fit it Together?* (Washington, D.C.: USGPO no. 053–003–00255–8, December 1976), p. iv.

2. Washington Business Group on Health: "A Private Sector Perspective on the Problems of Health Care Costs," working paper prepared for the Honorable Joseph Califano, Secretary, Department of Health, Education, and Welfare, Washington, D.C., April 1977.

3. Ashford, Nicholas A.: *Crisis in the Workplace: Occupational Disease and Injury* (Cambridge, Mass.: MIT Press, 1976), p. 4.

4. Ginzberg, Eli: "Health Services, Power Centers, and Decision-Making Mechanisms," *Daedalus* 106: 209 (Winter 1977).

5. Council on Wage and Price Stability, p. 77.

6. Lave, Judith R., Presentation at Cornell Conference for Business Executives, Ithaca, N.Y., May 1977.

7. Washington Business Group on Health, p. ii.

8. American Public Health Association: *Health and Work in America: A Chart Book* (Washington, D.C., November 1975), p. 107.

9. Samuels, Sheldon W.: "A Labor View of Company Medical Roles," in Lusterman, Seymour (ed.): *Health-Care Issues for Industry* (New York, Conference Board, 1974), p. 31.

Chapter 2. Industry as Payer

Assuming a Broader Role

1. Somers, Herman M., and Anne R. Somers: *Doctors, Patients, and Health Insurance* (Washington, D.C.: Brookings Institution, October 1967), p. 230.

2. Health Insurance Institute: *Source Book of Health Insurance Data, 1976–1977* (New York, 1977), p. 8.

3. Law, Sylvia A.: *Blue Cross, What Went Wrong?* (New Haven: Yale University Press, 1976), p. 6.

4. Ibid., p. 7.

5. Ibid., p. 10.

6. Krizay, John, and Andrew Wilson: *The Patient As Consumer* (Lexington, Mass.: Lexington Books, 1974).

7. Weeks, David A.: *National Health Insurance and Benefit Plans* (New York: Conference Board, 1974), p. 36.

8. Somers and Somers, p. 232.

9. United Mine Workers of America: Testimony Before the U.S. Senate Sub-Committee on Health and Scientific Research, Washington, D.C., May 31, 1977.

10. Weeks, p. 37.

11. Weeks, pp. 36–37.

12. *Employee Benefit Plan Review*, Chicago, no. 12 (June 1977), pp. 35–36.

13. Somers and Somers, chapter 12, pp. 228–246.

14. Krizay and Wilson, p. 6.

15. Law, p. 9.

16. Krizay and Wilson, chapter 3, pp. 37–50.

17. Somers and Somers, p. 231.

18. Council on Wage and Price Stability, p. 83.

19. Fuchs, Victor R.: *Who Shall Live?* (New York: Basic Books, 1974).

20. Council on Wage and Price Stability, p. 89.

An Expanding Benefit Package

1. Meyer, Mitchell, and Harland Fox: *Profile of Employee Benefits* (New York: Conference Board, 1974), p. 1.

2. Council on Wage and Price Stability, p. 84.

3. Chamber of Commerce of the United States: *Employee Benefits, 1975* (Washington, D.C., 1976).

4. Meyer and Fox, chapters 2 and 3, pp. 10–35.

5. U.S. Department of Health, Education, and Welfare, Public Health Service: *Forward Plan for Health, 1978–1982* (Washington, D.C.: USGPO no. 017–000–00172–8, August 1976), p. 31.

6. *Employee Benefit Plan Review*, Chicago, no. 12 (June 1977), pp. 8–9, 58.

7. Skolnik, Alfred M: "Twenty-Five Years of Employee Benefit Plans," *Social Security Bulletin* 3-21 (September 1976).

8. Skolnik, p. 12.

9. Krizay and Wilson, p. 33.

10. Council on Wage and Price Stability, p. 94.

Some Causes and Effects of Rising Costs

1. Klarman, Herbert E.: "The Financing of Health Care," Daedalus 106:215–234 (Winter 1977).

2. Council on Wage and Price Stability, p. 84.

3. Ibid.

4. Havighurst, Clark: "Controlling Health Care Costs: Strengthening the Private Sector's Hand," Journal of Health Politics, Policy and Law 1: 471–498 (1977).

5. Feldstein, Martin: "The High Costs of Hospitals and What to Do About It," The Public Interest 48: 40–54 (1977).

6. Roemer, Milton I., and Martin Shain: Hospital Utilization Under Insurance, Monograph Series, no. 6 (Chicago: American Hospital Association, 1959).

7. Wildavsky, Aaron: "Doing Better and Feeling Worse: The Political Pathology of Health Policy," Daedalus 106: 105–124 (Winter 1977).

8. Council on Wage and Price Stability, p. iii.

Approaches to Cost Containment

1. Washington Business Group on Health: "A Private Sector Perspective on the Problems of Health Care Costs," a working paper prepared for the Honorable Joseph Califano, Secretary, Department of Health, Education, and Welfare, Washington, D.C., April 1977, p. 10.

2. Washington Business Group on Health, p. 16.

3. Ibid., p. 20.

4. Somers, Anne R., and Herman M. Somers: "A Proposed Framework for Health and Health Care Policies," Inquiry 14: 115–170 (1977), p. 165.

5. Washington Business Group on Health, p. 10.

6. Council on Wage and Price Stability, p. 131.

7. Ibid., p. 24.

8. Ibid., p. 112.

9. Havighurst, Clark: "Controlling Health Care Costs: Strengthening the Private Sector's Hand," Journal of Health Politics, Policy and Law 1: 471–498 (1977).

10. Krizay, John, and Andrew Wilson: The Patient As Consumer (Lexington, Ma. Lexington Books, 1974), p. 66.

11. Council on Wage and Price Stability, p. 37.

12. Beck, R. G.: "The Effects of Copayment on the Poor," Journal of Human Resources 11 (Winter 1974).

13. Scitovsky, Anne A., and Nelda M. Snyder: "Effect of Coinsurance on Use of Physician Services," Social Security Bulletin 3-12 (June 1972).

14. Scitovsky, Anne A., and Nelda McCall: "Coinsurance and the Demand for Physician Services: Four Years Later," Social Security Bulletin 19-27 (May 1977).

15. Klarman, p. 226.

16. Hall, Charles P.: "Deductibles in Health Insurance: An Evaluation," Journal of Risk and Insurance, June 1966, p. 256.

17. Personal Communication, William J. Bicknell, M.D., Medical Director, United Mine Workers of America Health and Retirement Funds, August 1977.

18. Starr, Paul: "The Undelivered Health System," The Public Interest 42: 66–85, 1976.

19. Kirsch, Peter A.: "1976 HMO Amendments Will Aid Growth of Prepaid Care," *Public Health Reports* 92(2): 193–194 (1977).

20. Institute of Medicine: *Assessing Quality in Health Care: An Evaluation* (Washington, D.C.: IOM publication 76-04, November 1976).

21. Kraus, William A.: "PSRO Update: Where We Stand Now," *American Medical News,* June 20, 1977.

22. Brook, Robert H., and Kathleen N. Williams: *Evaluation of the New Mexico Peer Review System, 1971–1973* (Santa Monica, Calif.: Rand Corporation, 1977).

23. Washington Business Group on Health, p. 27.

24. Washington Business Group on Health, p. 11.

25. Wennberg, John G., and Alan Gittelsohn: "Small Area Variations in Health Care Delivery," *Science* 182: 1102–1108 (1973).

26. Bunker, John P.: "Surgical Manpower: A Comparison of Operations and Surgeons in the United States, and in England and Wales," *New England Journal of Medicine* 282: 135–144 (1970).

27. Moore, Francis D.: Surgical Manpower: Statistical Overview and Distributional Study. *Surgery in the United States:* A Summary Report of the Study on Surgical Services for the United States (Baltimore: American College of Surgeons–American Surgical Association, 1975).

28. Nickerson, Rita J., et al: "Doctors Who Perform Operations," *New England Journal of Medicine* 295: 921–926, 982–989 (1976).

29. Council on Wage and Price Stability, p. 109.

30. Washington Business Group on Health, p. 29.

31. Bogue, Ted: "Why Not the Most? A Physician's Guide to Locating in Cities With the Most Excessive Medicare Fees in the Country and an HEW Guide to Stopping this Waste of a Billion Dollars," Washington, D.C., Health Research Group, February 17, 1977.

32. Bauer, Katharine G.: "Hospital Rate Setting: This Way to Salvation?" *Milbank Memorial Fund Quarterly* 55: 117–158 (1977).

33. Council on Wage and Price Stability, p. 155.

34. Washington Business Group on Health, pp. 31–32.

Chapter 3. Industry as Provider

Early History

1. Somers, Anne R., and Herman M. Somers: *Doctors, Patients, and Health Insurance* (Washington, D.C.: Brookings Institution, 1961), p. 230.

2. Berman, Daniel M.: "Workers' Compensation," *Health PAC Bulletin* 71:9–14 (July–August 1976).

3. Ashford, Nicholas A.: *Crisis in the Workplace: Occupational Disease and Injury* (Cambridge, Mass.: MIT Press, 1976).

4. Smith, Robert Stewart: *The Occupational Safety and Health Act: Its Goals and Achievements* (Washington, D.C.: American Enterprise Institute for Public Policy Research, 1976), p. 29.

5. Barth, Peter S.: "The Effort to Rehabilitate Workers' Compensation," *American Journal of Public Health* 66: 553–557 (1976).

6. Hardy, Harriet L.: "Annual Discourse: Risk and Responsibility," *New England Journal of Medicine* 293: 801–806 (1975).

7. Blum, John D.: "Growing Legal Liability in Corporate Health Clinics," *Background Papers on Industry's Changing Role in Health Care Delivery*, Springer Series on Industry and Health Care, no. 3, p. 164 (1977).

8. Berman, p. 13.

9. Smith, p. 29.

10. Barth, p. 556.

11. Smith, p. 33.

12. U.S. Department of Labor, Occupational Safety and Health Review Commission, and U.S. Department of Health, Education, and Welfare: *The President's Report on Occupational Safety and Health* (Washington, D.C.: USGPO no. 040–000–00363–1, 1974), pp. 15–16, 115.

13. Navarro, Vincente: "The Underdevelopment of Health of Working America: Causes, Consequences, and Possible Solutions," *American Journal of Public Health* 66: 538–547 (1976).

14. *President's Report on Occupational Safety and Health*, 1974, p. 109.

15. Hiatt, Howard A.: "Protecting the Medical Commons: Who is Responsible?" *New England Journal of Medicine* 293: 235–241 (1975).

Occupational Medicine Takes Shape

1. Hanlon, John J.: *Public Health: Administration and Practice*, 6th ed. (St. Louis: Mosby, 1974), pp. 576–585.

2. Glasser, Melvin A.: "Workers' Health" *American Journal of Public Health*, 66: 529–530 (1976).

3. Samuels, Sheldon: "The Problems of Industry Sponsored Health Programs." *Background Papers on Industry's Changing Role in Health Care Delivery*, Springer Series on Industry and Health Care, no. 3, p. 152 (1977).

4. Hussey, R., quoted in Hanlon, p. 577.

5. Lusterman, Seymour: *Industry Roles in Health Care* (New York: Conference Board, 1974), pp. 15–16.

6. Quoted in Lusterman, p. 16.

7. Ashford, Nicholas A.: *Crisis in the Workplace: Occupational Disease and Injury* (Cambridge, Mass.: MIT Press, 1976).

8. Warshaw, Leon: "Industry's Role in the Delivery of Health Care," *Journal of Occupational Medicine* 13: 418–421 (1971).

9. Glasser, p. 530.

10. Corn, Morton: "OSHA Response to Occupational Health Personnel Needs and Resources," *American Industrial Hygiene Journal* 38: 11–17 (1977).

11. Ashford, chapter 9, pp. 424–475.

12. Block, Duane L. "Postgraduate Training of Occupational Physicians," *Journal of Occupational Medicine* 18: 755 (1976).

13. American Medical Association, Council on Occupational Health: "Physicians Guide to the Occupational Safety and Health Act of 1970," *Journal of the American Medical Association* 219: 905–907 (1972).

14. Hanlon, p. 577.

The Occupational Safety and Health Act

1. Smith, Robert Stewart: *The Occupational Safety and Health Act: Its Goals and Achievements* (Washington, D.C.: American Enterprise Institute for Public Policy Research, 1976), p. 5.

2. Ashford, Nicholas A. *Crisis in the Workplace: Occupational Disease and Injury* (Cambridge, Mass.: MIT Press, 1976).

3. Page, Joseph A., and Mary-Win O'Brien: *Bitter Wages: Ralph Nader's Study Group Report on Disease and Injury on the Job* (New York: Grossman, 1973).

4. Smith, *The Occupational Safety and Health Act* (1976).

5. U.S. Department of Labor, Occupational Safety and Health Review Commission, and U.S. Department of Health, Education, and Welfare: *The President's Report on Occupational Safety and Health* (Washington, D.C.: USGPO no. 040–000–00363–1, 1974), pp. 10–11.

6. Ashford, p. 3.

7. American Medical Association, Council on Occupational Health: "Physicians Guide to the Occupational Safety and Health Act of 1970," *Journal of the American Medical Association* 219: 906 (1972).

8. Ashford, p. 21.

9. Lusterman, Seymour: *Industry Roles in Health Care* (New York: Conference Board, 1974), pp. 15–16.

10. Lusterman, p. 13.

11. Somers, Herman M., and Anne R. Somers: *Doctors, Patients, and Health Insurance* (Washington, D.C.: Brookings Institution, October 1967), p. 230.

Industrial Medical Programs

1. Washington Business Group on Health: "A Private Sector Perspective on the Problems of Health Care Costs," working paper prepared for the Honorable Joseph Califano, Secretary, Department of Health Education, and Welfare, Washington, D.C., April 1977, p. 13.

2. Collings, Gilbeart H.: "Multiphasic Screening in the Occupational Health Setting," *Bulletin of the New York Academy of Medicine* 52: 517–527 (1976).

3. Cherry, William A., and Joseph Thomas Hamrick: "The Role of Automated Multiphasic Health Testing Services in Industrial Medicine," *Southern Medical Journal* 64: 929–934 (1971).

4. Breslow, Lester, and Anne R. Somers: "The Lifetime Health Monitoring Program," *New England Journal of Medicine* 296: 601–608 (1977).

5. Lewis, Hallet A.: "Determining the Cost Effectiveness of Occupational Health Programs," in Lusterman, Seymour (ed.): *Health-Care Issues for Industry* (New York: Conference Board, 1974), pp. 27–30.

6. Weinstein, Milton C., and William B. Stason: "Foundations of Cost-Effectiveness Analysis for Health and Medical Practices," *New England Journal of Medicine* 296: 716–721 (1977).

7. Falk, I. S.: "Medical Care: Its Social and Organizational Aspects: Labor Unions and Medical Care," *New England Journal of Medicine* 270: 22–28 (1964).

8. Herriman, Thomas: "Union Health Clinics," *Background Papers on Industry's Changing Role in Health Care Delivery*, Springer Series on Industry and Health Care, no. 3, p. 40 (1977).

9. Ibid.

10. Chamberlain, R. W., and J. F. Radebaugh: "Delivery of Primary Health Care—Union Style," *New England Journal of Medicine* 294: 641–645 (1976).

11. Lusterman, Seymour: *Industry Roles in Health Care* (New York: Conference Board, 1974).

12. Seubold, Frank H.: "HMOs: The View from the Program," *Public Health Reports* 90: 99–103 (1975).

13. Ellwood, Paul M., Jr., et al.: "Health Maintenance Strategy," *Medical Care* 9: 291–298 (1971).

14. Egdahl, Richard H.: "Foundations for Medical Care," *New England Journal of Medicine* 288: 491–498 (1973).

15. Gaus, Clifton R., Barbara S. Cooper, and Constance G. Hirshman: "Contrasts in HMO and Fee-for-Service Performance," *Social Security Bulletin* 3–14 (May 1976).

16. Egdahl, Richard H., et al.: "The Potential of Organizations of Fee-for-Service Physicians for Achieving Significant Decreases in Hospitalization," *Annals of Surgery* 186: 156–167 (1977).

17. Dorsey, Joseph L.: "Prepaid Group Practice and the Delivery of Ambulatory Care," *New England Journal of Medicine* 291(7) (1974).

18. Somers, Anne R. (ed.): *The Kaiser-Permanente Medical Care Program: A Symposium* (New York: Commonwealth Fund, 1971).

19. Lusterman, pp. 83–90.

20. Starr, Paul: "The Undelivered Health System," *Public Interest* 42: 66–85 (1976).

21. Kirsch, Peter A.: "1976 HMO Amendments Will Aid Growth of Prepaid Care," *Public Health Reports* 92(2): 193–194 (1977).

22. "Containing the Cost of Employee Benefit Plans," *Business Week*, May 30, 1977, pp. 74–76.

23. Lusterman, pp. 77–83.

24. See, for example, de Lisser, Stanley P.: "Contracting with an Independent Medical Organization for Corporate Health Programs," *Background Papers on Industry's Changing Role in Health Care Delivery*, Springer Series on Industry and Health Care, no. 3, p. 112 (1977).

25. Collings, Gilbeart H.: "Health—A Corporate Dilemma: Health Care Management—A Corporate Solution," *Background Papers on Industry's Changing Role in Health Care Delivery*, Springer Series on Industry and Health Care, no. 3, p. 16 (1977).

26. Egdahl, Richard H., and Diana Chapman Walsh: "Industry–Sponsored Health Programs: Basis for a New Hybrid Prepaid Plan," *New England Journal of Medicine* 296: 1350–1353 (1977).

Chapter 4. Industry as Consumer

Community Health Planning

1. Vladeck, Bruce C.: "Interest-Group Representation and the HSAs," *American Journal of Public Health* 67: 23–29 (1977).

2. Lusterman, Seymour: "A Partnership for Business in Health Care?" *Conference Board Record*, October 1972, pp. 24–27.

3. Blendon, Robert J.: "The Changing Role of Private Philanthropy in Health Affairs," *New England Journal of Medicine* 292: 946–950 (1975).

4. Somers, Herman M.: "Health and Public Policy." *Inquiry* 12(2): 87–96 (1975).

5. Sieverts, Stephen: *Health Planning Issues and Public Law 93-641* (Chicago, American Hospital Association, 1977).

6. Werlin, Stanley H., Alexandra Walcott, and Michael Joroff: "Implementing Formative Health Planning under P.L. 93–641," *New England Journal of Medicine* 295:698–703 (1976).

7. Sieverts, p. 81.

8. Bicknell, William J., and Diana Chapman Walsh: "Critical Experiences in Organizing and Administering a State Certificate of Need Program," *Public Health Reports* 91: 29–45 (1976).

9. Walsh, Diana Chapman, and William J. Bicknell: "Forecasting the Need for Hospital Beds: A Quantitative Methodology," *Public Health Reports* 92: 199–210 (1977).

10. Werlin, Walcott, Joroff, p. 699.

11. Sieverts, 14–19.

Industry Involvement in Health Planning

1. Ellwood, Paul M., Jr.: "Business and the Changing Health-Care Scene," in Lusterman, Seymour (ed.): *Health-Care Issues for Industry* (New York: Conference Board, 1974), pp. 53–60.

2. Washington Business Group on Health: "A Private Sector Perspective on the Problems of Health Care Costs," working paper prepared for the Honorable Joseph Califano, Secretary, Department of Health Education, and Welfare, Washington, D.C., April 1977, p. 24.

3. Executive Office of the President, Council on Wage and Price Stability *The Complex Puzzle of Rising Health Care Costs: Can the Private Sector Fit it Together?* (Washington, D.C.: USGPO no. 053–003–00255, December 1976), pp. 131–135.

4. Goldbeck, Willis B.: "Health Planning: An Essential Ingredient in Cost Containment," *National Journal,* June 4, 1977, pp. 876–877.

5. Washington Business Group on Health, pp. A–2, A–3.

6. Rice, Judith: "General Motors Attacks Rising Health Costs," *Modern Healthcare,* September, 1976, pp. 14–15.

7. Washington Business Group on Health, pp. A–9, A–10.

8. Council on Wage and Price Stability, p. 171.

9. Miller, Gay Sands: "Beds and Boards: Agencies Act to Lower Health Bills by Saying No to Bigger Hospitals," *Wall Street Journal,* May 5, 1977, p. 1.

10. Washington Business Group on Health, p. 7.

11. Ibid., p. 28.

12. McClure, Walter: "Reducing Excess Hospital Capacity," prepared for Bureau of Health Planning and Resources Development, Department of Health, Education, and Welfare (contract no. HRA-230–76–0086), October 15, 1976, p. 66.

13. Washington Business Group on Health, pp. A–4, A–7.

14. Institute of Medicine: *Controlling the Supply of Hospital Beds* (Washington, D.C.: National Academy of Sciences, publication no. 0–309–02610–5, October 1976).

15. McClure, p. 1.

16. McClure, p. iv.

17. Council on Wage and Price Stability, pp. 72–73.

18. Somers, p. 164.

19. Griffith, John R., Walton M. Hancock, and Fred C. Munson: "Practical Ways to Contain Hospital Costs," Harvard Business Review, November-December, 1973, pp. 131–139.

20. Griffith, John R., Walton M. Hancock, and Fred C. Munson: Cost Control in Hospitals (Ann Arbor, Mich.: Health Administration Press, 1976).

21. Washington Business Group on Health, p. 29.

Individual Decisions about Health and Health Care

1. Lalonde, Marc: A New Perspective on the Health of Canadians (Ottawa: Department of National Health and Welfare, April 1974).

2. Ibid., p. 15.

3. U.S. Department of Health, Education, and Welfare, Public Health Service: Forward Plan for Health, 1977–1981 (Washington, D.C.: DHEW publication no. [05] 76–50024, August 1975).

4. U.S. Department of Health, Education, and Welfare, p. 98.

5. Barclay, W. R.: "Hypertension: A Major Medical Care Challenge," Journal of the American Medical Association 235: 2327 (1976).

6. Alderman, Michael M., and Ellie E. Schoenbaum: "Detection and Treatment of Hypertension at the Work Site," New England Journal of Medicine 293: 65–68 (1975).

7. Knowles, John H.: "The Responsibility of the Individual," Daedalus 106: 57–80 (Winter 1977).

8. Ogden, Horace G.: "Health Education: A Federal Overview," Public Health Reports 91: 199–205 (1976).

9. Somers, Anne R., and Herman M. Somers: "Proposed Framework for Health and Health Care Policies," Inquiry 14: 115–170 (1977), p. 130.

10. Lave, Judith R., and Lester B. Lave: "Measuring the Effectiveness of Prevention, I," Milbank Memorial Fund Quarterly 55: 273–290 (1977).

11. Shapiro, Sam.: "Measuring the Effectiveness of Prevention, II," Milbank Memorial Fund Quaterly 55: 291–306 (1977).

Chapter 5. Summing Up

1. Executive Office of the President, Council on Wage and Price Stability The Complex Puzzle of Rising Health Care Costs: Can the Private Sector Fit it Together? (Washington, D.C.: USGPO no. 053–003–00255–8, December 1976), pp. iiv–iv.

2. Butler, Robert N.: Why Survive? Being Old in America (New York: Harper and Row, 1975).

3. Manney, James D., Jr.: Aging in American Society: An Examination of Concepts and Issues (Ann Arbor, Mich.: University of Michigan, 1975).

4. Brotman, Herman B. "The Fastest Growing Minority: The Aged," American Journal of Public Health 64: 249–252 (1974).

5. U.S. Department of Health, Education, and Welfare, Public Health Service: Health: United States, 1975 (Rockville, Md.: DHEW publication no. [HRA] 76–1232, 1976).

Chapter 6. Issues for the Future

1. Fuchs, Victor: *Who Shall Live?* (New York: Basic Books, 1974).

2. Carlson, Rick I.: *The End of Medicine* (New York: John Wiley, 1975).

3. Knowles, John H.: "The Responsibility of the Individual," *Daedalus* 106: 57–80 (Winter 1977).

4. Hiatt, Howard H.: "Protecting the Medical Commons: Who is Responsible?" *New England Journal of Medicine* 293: 235–241 (1975).

5. Reinhardt, Uwe E.: "Future Perspectives on the Problem: Where Will We be in Five Years," in *Controlling Health Care Costs: A National Leadership Conference* (National Journal: Washington, D.C., in press).

Annotated Bibliography

Alderman, Michael H., M.D., and Ellie F. Schoenbaum. "Detection and Treatment of Hypertension at the Worksite." *New England Journal of Medicine,* vol. 293, no. 2 (July 10, 1975), pp. 65–68.

A union-offered program to identify and treat asymptomatic, uncomplicated hypertension is described. Key elements of the program are "provision of all diagnostic and therapeutic services at the worksite, delivery of care within a cohesive union structure, adherence to a rigid protocol, and continuous patient surveillance by nurses and paraprofessionals under physician supervision." Of the nearly 100 union members who entered the program, 81% achieved reductions in diastolic blood pressure of at least 10%. The authors conclude "that this occupationally based, systematic method of hypertension control is acceptable, safe, and effective.

Ashford, Nicholas A. *Crisis in the Workplace: Occupational Disease and Injury.* MIT Press, Cambridge, Mass., 1976.

A "voluminous" report on the state of occupational health and safety in the United States; the extent of the "crisis"; how the problem has been, and is being, addressed by government, management, labor, and special interest groups; and the scientific-technical, legal, political, and economic problems which impact on both the problem and our capability to deal with it. Also included are foreign experiences in worker safety and health, and a series of governmental and private sector policy recommendations.

Bauer, Katharine G. "Hospital Rate Setting—This Way to Salvation?" *Health and Society (MMFQ)*, vol. 55, no. 1 (Winter 1977), pp. 117–158.

  The factors giving rise to hospital rate setting programs; the different approaches that have been, and are being, attempted; the various specific objectives of rate-setting programs; the methods of determining rates and the knowledge and information gaps impacting on them; the designed and accidental risks inherent in rate setting programs; and the structural and behavioral incentives and disincentives for cost control set in motion by various rate-setting approaches are all reviewed by Bauer. She argues that, in the absence of a broader policy of health regulation, and without appropriate linkages between rate setting and planning, utilization review, and quality assurance programs, expectations for real cost containment through rate setting should be modest.

Brook, Robert H. and Kathleen N. Williams. "Evaluation of the New Mexico Peer Review System 1971 to 1973." *Medical Care*, vol. 14, no. 12 (December 1976), Supplement.

  Primarily an analysis of the performance of the New Mexico EMCRO (Experimental Medical Care Review Organization) in controlling costs and assuring the quality of medical services provided Medicaid beneficiaries, this work also includes a short overview of evaluative studies on other PSRO prototypes. The program resulted in gross savings (implicit and explicit) of 15% of the amount billed by providers, but only 13% of these savings were attributable to direct denials (3%) or implicit savings (10%), and the likelihood of larger savings' being realized "is small unless nursing home and (especially) hospital utilization can be controlled."

Chamberlin, R. W., M.D., and J. F. Radebaugh, M.D. "Delivery of Primary Health Care—Union Style." *New England Journal of Medicine*, vol. 294, no. 12 (March 18, 1976), pp. 641–645.

  The authors review the genesis of a network of primary care clinics operated by the United Farm Workers of America. Unlike many other employee benefit programs, this program is "designed for workers who are without employment for weeks at a time." It has also been innovative in a number of areas (outreach, clinic location and hours, health education and concern about living conditions, etc.) that have markedly increased its usefulness to the members. However, the authors note that the complete consumer control of the health clinics has resulted in poor working conditions and high staff turnover. They conclude that "complete consumer control has built into it the same hazards as complete professional control."

Egdahl, Richard H., M.D. "Foundations for Medical Care." *New England Journal of Medicine*, vol. 288, no. 10 (March 8, 1973), pp. 491–498.

  The origins and diversity of Foundations for Medical Care (FMCs), where participating physicians are reimbursed in direct proportion to the services they provide, are reviewed. FMCs have demonstrated an ability to produce cost savings and quality control through claims review, peer review, fee schedules, and (in the more comprehensive models) such tools as utilization controls and financial risk involvement by the participating physicians.

Ehrbar, A. F. "A Radical Prescription for Medical Care." *Fortune*, February 1977, pp. 164–170, 172.

  The range of national health insurance proposals to date would basically extend the type of insurance coverage that most people already have to more people, or transfer all payment responsibilities to the federal government. Either is likely to trigger a rapid increase in demands with resulting increases in either costs or (under the latter approach) other rationing mechanisms such as delays in service. Ehrbar proposes releasing the "invisible hand" of the market in health care: most consumers would opt for higher deductible and catastrophic coverage (which could be provided by the federal government) and accept the risk for a reasonable level of medical expenses themselves (or join health maintenance organizations and shift some of the risks and incentives to the providers).

Ellwood, Paul M., Jr., and Michael E. Herbert. "Health Care: Should Industry Buy It or Sell It?" *Harvard Business Review*, vol. 51, no. 4 (July–August 1973), pp. 99–107.

The authors characterize the U.S. health industry as beset by "uninformed consumers, a lack of management skills, small and fragmented delivery units, noncompetitive cost-plus pricing features, and inefficient incentives for both the buyers and sellers of health services." Reforms that will return the market function to the health sector are suggested, including corporate investment in health maintenance organizations. A series of questions that any company pondering whether to step into the HMO field should consider are listed. If the decision is reached to proceed, a number of strategy concepts are discussed. Potential returns on investment from sound and profitable HMO management are discussed.

Executive Office of the President, Council on Wage and Price Stability. *The Rapid Rise of Hospital Costs*. U.S. Government Printing Office, Washington, D.C., 1977. Publication no. 725–155–752.

This report isolates and investigates the forces that have caused hospital costs to increase at a rate that exceeds those observed for all major contributors to total health care costs. The study determines that the historically observed hospital cost increase is the inherent result of the structure and financing of the hospital industry, particularly insurance coverage, and "nothing short of fundamental reforms or alterations of this structure will cause the inflationary pressure to abate."

Fuchs, Victor R. *Who Shall Live?* Basic Books, New York, 1974.

Subtitled "Health, Economics, and Social Choice," this book notes the contributions, and limitations, which economics can provide to our understanding of the health care problems (e.g., cost, accessibility, and concern about insufficient health status). It documents that medical care, despite its rapidly increasing cost, has only a relatively small influence on health status in comparison with nonmedical factors such as pollution, lifestyles, and water fluoridation. Economic analysis can give direction to health policy considerations, such as the potential for controlling expenditures, but the author warns of the critical importance of value choices which are "at the root of most of our major health problems."

Greenberg, Ira G., and Michael L. Rodburg. "The Role of Prepaid Group Practice in Relieving the Medical Care Crisis." *Harvard Law Review*, vol. 84, no. 4 (February 1971), pp. 889–1001.

Common perceptions of many of the aspects of the "medical care crisis" have undergone considerable redefinition and change of emphasis since the early 1970s when this article was written. Nevertheless, there is value in reviewing the nature of the environment faced by prepaid group plans a relatively short time ago to appreciate the speed of change. In addition, many of the factors discussed in this article are still timely: among them are PPGP principles of operation, various PPGP-hospital relationships, sources of economic savings, and issues affecting the attractiveness of PPGPs to both consumers and providers.

Griffith, John R., Walton M. Hancock, and Fred C. Munson. "Practical Ways to Contain Hospital Costs." *Harvard Business Review,* November–December 1973, pp. 131–139.

Based on four years of study at two medium-sized hospitals in Michigan, the authors recommend a number of strategies that trustees of hospitals can adopt to encourage effective controls on hospital costs: encourage and support community-wide planning (so economies implemented at one hospital are not "offset by expenditures at a neighboring institution") and tight control over bed supply through certificate of need programs. Within their own hospitals, it is suggested that trustees ask more questions about cost/benefit justification for proposed expansions of services, encourage adoption of incentive or prospective reimbursement contracts with third parties, and provide strong support and rewards for management initiative toward cost control.

Havighurst, Clark. "Controlling Health Care Costs: Strengthening the Private Sector's Hand." *Journal of Health Politics, Policy and Law,* vol. 1 (1977), pp. 471–498.

Health delivery and cost control concerns of the American people can best be met through a diversity of private insurance initiatives. If freed of undue legal restrictions and organized provider resistance, private insurers could pursue a range of cost-control measures, such as required second opinions and higher deductible policies, that would place many decisions back in the hands of cost-conscious consumers. This would encourage doctors to compete on the basis of achieving results at less cost rather than, as at present, by providing more services.

Hiatt, Howard H., M.D. "Protecting the Medical Commons: Who is Responsible?" *NEJM,* vol. 293 (July 31, 1975), pp. 235–241.

Likening the total resources society can allocate for medical care, research, and teaching to the "common," or town pasture, of time gone-by, Hiatt argues that we are rapidly approaching a state of "overgrazing" which if continued will result in the eventual ruin of the common. It would be inappropriate and unfair of society to leave to physicians alone the responsibility of developing new priorities for access to our medical resources; consumers, politicians, economists, and many other groups also need to be involved. Hiatt indicates several guidelines: funds should be set aside for basic research and the training of researchers, the public must be educated about their own bodies and the limits of medical intervention, and the decision-making process must be flexible enough to adjust to rapidly changing conditions.

Krizay, John, and Andrew Wilson. *The Patient As Consumer.* Lexington Books, Lexington, Mass., 1974.

This book explores whether the private insurance industry has "the motivation or the means to control the quality and cost of health care, and whether it can contribute to the efficiency and quality of a universal health care system" if adopted. The authors conclude that "while the private sector insurers have borne much of the criticism for the deficiencies of the health care system and medical care inflation, . . . the public sector . . . has had an even greater opportunity to exert an influence [over these deficiencies]." In addition to a discussion of necessary health insurance reforms, readers can find basic information on a wide number of topics, including the workings of the health insurance industry (profits, benefits, accounting procedures, incentives, etc.); insurance influences on demand for and supply of hospital and physician services, prices, costs, and utilization, and how these influences can be modified by cost-sharing arrangements; and a discussion of real and imagined advantages of prepaid group practices.

Lalonde, Marc. *A New Perspective on the Health of Canadians.* Department of National Health and Welfare, Ottawa, Canada, 1974.

Although the health status of the Canadian people has risen as the result of improvements in health care, standard of living, public health, and medical science, their health is now threatened by some of the consequences of the economic progress that contributed to earlier improvements. These threats to health status include environmental (pollution) and behavioral (abuse of alcohol, tobacco and other drugs, overindulgent eating and malnutrition, etc.) forces for which the traditional health care system is not well-organized to effectively intervene except after the avoidable damage to the individual's health has already occurred. Lalonde concludes that "further improvements in the environment, reductions in self-imposed risks, and a greater knowledge of human biology are necessary if more Canadians are to live a full, happy, long, and illness-free life."

Lusterman, Seymour. *Industry Roles in Health Care.* The Conference Board, New York, 1974. Report No. 610.

This report is an analysis of survey responses from a sample of manufacturing, transportation, utilization, wholesale/retail, financial, and other large industries (employing 500 or more persons) on their internal (preemployment and placement exams, health education, in-house or contractual occupational and nonoccupational health services for employees, staffing of health services, environmental surveillance, periodic screening, etc.) and external (community-wide planning, health maintenance organization development, providing health services to nonemployees, legislative support, etc.) involvement in health care. Many, but not a majority, of the responding companies have expanded their health care activities during the ten-year period prior to this survey, but very few are found to have reevaluated the "traditional relationships between company medical departments and the wider health care system, or to be taking on more active community roles than in the past."

McCarthy, Eugene G., M.D., and Geraldine W. Widmer, R.N. "Effects of Screening by Consultants on Recommended Elective Surgical Procedures." *New England Journal of Medicine,* vol. 291, no. 25 (December 19, 1974), pp. 1331–1335.

Too much unnecessary surgery and hospitalization occurs in the United States, yet surgical care is traditionally monitored retrospectively. McCarthy and Widmer report on the experience of two union groups that have adopted a second surgical opinion program. Over a two-year period, consultants failed to confirm the necessity of hospitalization in 21% and 31% of the cases. Program operating costs were only about one-eighth of the estimated savings from hospital admissions not made and surgical procedures not performed, but these estimates and "the findings of this report should be considered preliminary."

McClure, Walter. *Reducing Excess Hospital Capacity.* Bureau of Health Planning and Resources Development, Department of Health, Education, and Welfare, October 15, 1976. Contract no. HRA—230-76-0086.

Our current hospital capacity is excessive in terms of both excess idle capacity and our unnecessary utilization of these expensive resources. Citing supportive evidence including low average occupancy, the correlation (within typical ranges of hospital utilization) of higher hospital utilization with more hospital capacity rather than health status, widespread peer review findings of unnecessary admissions and patients kept hospitalized beyond the time required medically, hospital utilization among comparable populations varying by as much as 300%, and studies confirming that health maintenance organizations providing care of equal effectiveness as the fee-for-service system are able to cut hospital utilization 30–50%, McClure concludes that substantial reductions in hospital capacity (and costs) can be made without harming the welfare of the public.

Meyer, Mitchell, and Harland Fox. *Profile of Employee Benefits.* The Conference Board, New York, 1974. (Report No. 645.)

Based on a comparison to a similar, though more limited, survey made in the early 1960s, this report presents current characteristics and coverage trends in employee benefits packages as indicated by returns from nearly 1800 businesses to a Conference Board survey undertaken in 1972–1973. Major trends observed include increased uniformity of benefits for all employees of the same company (attributed primarily to growing union power, the economic advantages available when requiring fewer insurance policies for more workers, and government regulations requiring wider eligibility for benefits in many trusted benefit funds); increases, in each of the benefit areas, in the proportion of companies providing benefits to employees on a noncontributory basis (attributed to unionism and company paternalism); a decrease in the level of new innovations in benefit programs; and increased government intervention and regulation of employee benefits.

Newhouse, Joseph P., Charles E. Phelps, and William B. Schwartz, M.D. "Policy Options and the Impact of National Health Insurance." *New England Journal of Medicine,* vol. 290, no. 24 (June 13, 1974), pp. 1345–1359.

Three policy issues are examined concerning national health insurance: "How much change in demand for health services will be created by any given insurance program and how much will such a change alter the nations' health care bill?"; "How readily can each component of the health-delivery system respond to the anticipated increase in demand, and what will the consequences be if the demand for services cannot immediately be satisfied?"; and "How much improvement in the nation's health status can be anticipated in response to a new health insurance program?". The probable impact of each of the health-care financing proposals on these three issues is discussed. The appropriate structure of a national health insurance program will depend upon the goals established by society, and the authors provide several examples of how program design and goal determination interact.

Price, Daniel M. "Private Industry Health Insurance Plans: Types of Administration and Insurer in 1974." *Social Security Bulletin,* March 1977, pp. 13–27, 42.

A survey of health insurance provisions for private industry employees conducted by the Bureau of Labor Statistics provides information representing over 50,000 plans based on a sample of 1,600 plans. The three most important types of plans, in terms of percentage of workers covered, are employer-administered nonnegotiated plans (43%), employer-administered negotiated plans (32%), and joint worker-employer-administered negotiated plans (23%). "In general, workers in employer-administered negotiated plans were more likely to have basic hospital benefits, service benefits, or higher cash allowances, more days-in-hospital coverage, and basic surgical benefits and higher cash benefits than those in other plans, particularly those in nonnegotiated plans." In addition, since Blue Cross insurance is relatively most prevalent among employer-administered negotiated plans, "higher proportions of workers under Blue Cross plans had liberal benefit coverages than of workers insured otherwise."

Schultze, Charles L. "The Public Use of Private Interest." *Harpers*, May 1977, pp. 43–62.

Beginning with a review of the changing and growing nature of governmental regulation in the United States, Schultze underscores that once a political consensus has been reached to intervene, the extent and scope of the regulatory process are seldom based on an analysis of shortcomings in the private market on how the "imperfect" regulation process will result in better outcomes than the "imperfect" private market mechanisms it will replace. Secondly, due to historical and political characteristics, regulatory programs almost always are along the lines of eliminating characteristics (by implementing centralized regulatory bodies, providing free services, etc.) rather than modifying existing incentives so that parties acting in their own self-interest will also serve the broader social goals. Schultze sees substantial economic and social costs to our overreliance on regulatory "control and command," and argues that such efforts are often doomed to failure.

Skolnik, Alfred M. "Twenty-Five Years of Employee-Benefit Plans," *Social Security Bulletin*, September 1976, pp. 3–21.

Skolnik provides a statistical and a descriptive analysis of the major characteristics and trends observed in employee-benefit health and welfare funds from 1950 through 1974. The report is limited to programs sponsored or initiated by the employer and/or the employees, and which are not directly underwritten or paid for by government (such as Workers' Compensation). Contributions to health plans have increased sharply, from $850 million in 1950 to over $23 billion in 1974. Benefits during this same period grew from $708 million to over $21 billion and account for 50% of all benefits paid out under the different types of employee-benefit plans. Characteristics of health plans are also described, such as type of benefits offered, type of insurance organization used, and financing responsibilities assumed by employers and employees.

Smith, Robert Stewart. *The Occupational Safety and Health Act: Its Goals and Its Achievements.* American Enterprise Institute for Public Policy Research, Washington, D.C., 1976.

Smith "argues that the safety and health mandate of the Occupational Safety and Health Act of 1970 is inconsistent with the goal of promoting the general welfare." This conclusion is based on the view that the act requires expenditures for health and safety beyond the amount that workers would themselves choose to make if they paid for such efforts directly. It is suggested that the level of occupational injury could be reduced less expensively and more effectively by repealing safety standards and, since there is no evidence that the private market underprovides (in relation to the cost-benefit framework) occupational safety, simply instituting modest fines on employers for each occupational injury sustained by their employees.

Warshaw, Leon J., M.D. "Industry's Role in Health Care Delivery." *Journal of Occupational Medicine*, vol. 13, no. 10 (October 1973), pp. 790–792.

Warshaw presents his personal views about why industry is, or should be, becoming involved in health care, and the special resources industry can bring to improving health care delivery. Reasons range from self-interest (enhancing the functional integrity of its work force, meeting legal responsibilities, making money, containing the cost of employee health benefits, etc.) to moral and community obligations. The overwhelming reason, however, is that "industry can do it better!" Industry can bring management and marketing know-how, and capital for planning, implementation, and operational subsidization until break-even is reached. Warshaw rejects government except as a "desperate last resort."

Weeks, David A. *National Health Insurance and Corporate Benefit Plans.* The Conference Board, New York, 1974. Report no. 633.

This report examines the major probable effects of national health insurance implementation on corporate employee-benefit health plans. Although NHI would establish expanded minimum health insurance benefits, Weeks forsees only limited impact on employee-benefit plans as a result. More sweeping improvements in worker benefits would result if, as Week's expects, preventive services benefits are covered and NHI has the effect of increasing the rate at which currently innovative benefits (e.g., dental benefits and higher major medical limits) are added. Another suggested impact on businesses is that, with the abandonment of experience rating, corporations that have invested in in-house employee health programs will be effectively penalized as their per capita or payroll contributions to NHI increase.

Wennberg, John, M.D., and Alan Gittelshon "Small Area Variations in Health Care Delivery." *Science,* vol. 182 (December 14, 1973), pp. 1102–1108.

Variations in hospital, surgical, and ancillary service utilization rates among thirteen hospital service areas in Vermont are presented. Comparison of surgery rates and the number of physicians performing surgery within service areas showed a strong positive correlation. Age-adjusted annual hospital discharge rates varied between 122 and 197 per 1,000 persons, and hospital days utilized per 1,000 persons show a similar degree of spread. Medicare per capita (beneficiary) reimbursement for ancillary services varied by as much as 400% (diagnostic x-ray) to 700% (laboratory) among hospital service areas. These "variations in utilization indicate that there is considerable uncertainty about the effectiveness of different levels of aggregate, as well as specific kinds of, health services."